EPIDEMIOLOGY OF THE RISK FACTORS FOR CEREBROVASCULAR DISEASE

AUTHOR: ASSOCIATE PROFESSOR IVAN MANCHEV MD, PHD
TECHNICAL ASSISTANT: VASIL KALPACHEV, MD

authorHOUSE®

AuthorHouse™ UK Ltd.
500 Avebury Boulevard
Central Milton Keynes, MK9 2BE
www.authorhouse.co.uk
Phone: 08001974150

© 2010 Ivan Manchev, MD, PhD. All rights reserved.

No part of this book may be reproduced, stored in a retrieval system, or transmitted by any means without the written permission of the author.

First published by AuthorHouse 2/9/2010

ISBN: 978-1-4490-5507-3 (sc)

This book is printed on acid-free paper.

BOOK REVIEW

Despite considerable progress in the research on eatiopatogenesis, clinical manifestations, diagnosis and treatment of cardiovascular disease (CVD), its risk factors are still a matter of debate. The present book, written by the head of the Department of Neurology and Psychiatry of the Faculty of Medicine, Thracian University, Stara Zagora, Bulgaria, presents a brief overview of the major risk factors for CVD with particular reference to the local problems in his home country and based on personal investigations. After an introduction with classification of the risk factors for CVD, the well documented (arterial hypertension, cardiovascular diseases, smoking, carotid stenoses, diabetes, etc.) and less well documented ones (dyslipidemia, alcohol abusus obesity and others), epidemiological data from the literature are summarized for each of these risk factors. Results from personal population-based epidemiological studies of cerebrovascular risk factors in 500 Bulgarian subjects are presented. As presumed, cardiovascular disorders and diabetes mellitus were more frequent in the old compared with the young age groups, asymptomatic carotid artery stenoses prevailed in women of both age groups, smoking was frequent in both genders aged 50–59 years. Increased total cholesterol and LDL was more frequent in women, increased HDL in men, as was increased alcohol abuse. Combinations of two or more risk factors were observed in more than one-third of the investigated healthy individuals. Among these combinations prevailed hypertension, dyslipidemias, overweight, smoking and cardiovascular diseases, with a significant age-related increase of arterial hypertension, similar to the data of the Austrian and British populations. The incidences of cardiovascular diseases, diabetes mellitus and haemodynamically active carotid artery stenosis in the Bulgarian cohort was similar to those in other populations, and the incidence of hypercholesterolaemia and overweight likewise agreed with the results of other population-based epidemiological studies, while the incidence of some other risk factors for CVD differed from other populations. This first Bulgarian population-based study of risk factors for CVD in comparison to epidemiological studies in other populations are of interest for all who are concerned with risk factors of CVD and their prophylaxis.

Prof. K. A. Jellinger, MD
Director Institute of Clinical Neurology
Vienna, Austria

Contents

INTRODUCTION 1
I. Risk factors for cerebrovascular disease (CVD) 2
II. Classification of the RF for CVD 5
1. Well documented RF for CVD 6
1.1. Arterial hypertension 6
1.2. Cardiovascular diseases 8
1.2.1. Atrial fibrillation 9
1.2.2. Ischemic heart disease (IHD) 11
1.2.3. Left ventricular hypertrophy 13
1.3. Smoking 15
1.4. Asymptomatic carotid stenoses 17
1.5. Diabetes mellitus 19
1.6. Transient ischemic attacks 22
1.7. Other well documented risk factors 24
2. Less well documented risk factors 24
2.1 Dyslipidemies 24
2.2 Alcohol abuse 26
2.3 Reduced physical activity 27
2.4 Obesity 28
2.5. Increased hematocrit and fibrinogen 29
2.6. Other less well documented risk factors 31
III. Descriptive and analytical studies of RFs for CVD in our country 32
IV. Problems under discussion 34
V. PERSONAL INVESTIGATIONS 36
5.1. Results from population-based epidemiological study of
   Cerebrovascular risk factors 36
5.1.1. Arterial hypertension 36
5.1.2. Diseases of the cardiovascular system 43
5.1.2.1. Atrial fibrillation 43
5.1.2.2. Ischemic heart disease 43
5.1.2.3. Left ventricular hypertrophy 43
5.1.3. Smoking 46
5.1.4. Asymptomatic carotid stenoses 48
5.1.5. Diabetes mellitus 52
5.2. Less well documented risk factors for CVD 54
5.2.1. Hyperlipidemia 54
5.2.2. Use of oral contraceptives 60
5.2.3. Alcohol abuse 61
5.2.4. Obesity 63
5.2.5. Increased hematocrit 66

5.2.6. Reduced physical activity.. 67
5.2.7. Migraine 70
5.3. Combination of risk factors for CVD.. 71
5.4. The importance of electroencephalographic deviations for the
   assessment of the risk for acute cerebral circulatory disorder 77
SUMMARY 81
REFERENCES 85
ABBREVIATIONS USED IN THE MONOGRATH 108

INTRODUCTION

Despite of the progress achieved in the research of etiopathogenesis, clinical manifestation and diagnostics of cerebrovascular diseases (CVD), their treatment is not effective enough. It is, therefore, of great importance for the practice to identify, reveal and therapeutically affect the cerebrovascular risk factors (CRF) for CVD. A common definition for the term 'risk factor'(RF) is still missing. RF is not a direct cause for a particular disease but participates in complex and not always clarified relations to these causes. In general, RFs are defined as physiological peculiarities of a person as well as lifestyle and nutrition that increase the possibility of a certain disease development. On the other hand, although the presence of risk factors increases the possibility of disease development, it does not obligatory lead to its manifestation. The risk is measured by means of studying the morbidity in descriptive epidemiological studies. The basic indicators for measuring the risk are several.

The relative risk represents the ratio between morbidity and/or mortality of a certain disease among the individuals with one or several RFs compared to the control group of healthy individuals. From practical point of view it is important to know what will be the effect from elimination of the considered factor on the population. The so called attributive risk is used to measure this effect. The attributive risk characterizes the specific risk due to one causal factor. The attributive risk for the whole population is called population attributive risk and defined as the absolute difference between the risk and morbidity in the total population and the one in the non-exposed group. Options ratio (OR) is used in the epidemiological studies by the case-control method and the ratio between the morbidity option in the exposed group and the morbidity option in the non-exposed group is defined. A number of clinical-epidemiological studies demonstrated that arterial hypertension was the riskiest factor for ischemic and hemorrhagic disorders of the cerebral circulation. Cardiovascular diseases were on the second place of importance among the risk factors for stroke. The important role of atrial fibrillation, acute myocardial infarction and left ventricular hypertrophy was pointed out. The risk for cerebral infarction was increased in diabetic patients but it well correlated to the presence of arterial hypertension. It was found that smoking was an independent risk factor for cerebrovascular diseases and most of all for cerebral and subarachnoid hemorrhages. Currently, it was found that asymptomatic carotid stenoses which were hemodynamically significant led to development of cerebral infarction.

The role of less well documented risk factors for CVD provoked unarguable interest. It is known that hyperlipidemias are associated with atherosclerotic process progression in the coronary and cerebral arteries. The high serum concentrations of cholesterol, LDL and triglycerides and the decreased HDL arefavorable events for this. Overweight is also attributed to the probable risk factors for stroke.

Good knowledge of the different cerebrovascular risk factors gives the opportunity for effective primary and secondary prophylaxis of CVD. The following risk factors for cerebrovascular diseases belong to those that cannot be influenced: age, male gender, family predisposition, race, etc. Primary prophylaxis includes non-medicinal treatment which is directed to change in the lifestyle and medicinal treatment of the arterial hypertension, cardiovascular diseases, diabetes mellitus and hyperlipidemias. Secondary prophylaxis that is also medicinal and surgical aims to reduce the risk for relapses.

I. Risk factors for cerebrovascular disease (CVD)

Stroke is preceded by a number of pathologic processes and impairments that increase at different level the risk for its occurrence.

These are cerebrovascular risk factors (CRF) that are various and have big variety and different frequency in different geographic regions.

The project MONICA of WHO showed that stroke morbidity studied in 18 populations from Europe and Asia varied widely from 101 to 285 per 100, 000 men and from 40 to 198 per 100, 000 women. Parameters of morbidity increased when relapses of preceding strokes were included. Stroke morbidity and mortality were bigger in Eastern European countries than those in Western and North Europe (*Stegmeyer B et al. 1997*). Descriptive and epidemiological studies in Austria (*Vutung C et al. 1997*) and Spain (*Jover - Saenz A et al. 1999*) with the methods of multivariate logistic regression analysis showed that stroke morbidity significantly decreased in last years. Another big epidemiological study held in 22 European countries also showed bigger morbidity and mortality in Eastern Europe compared to Western countries (*Brainin M et al. 2000*). ERICA, another project of WHO, revealed that hypertension, hypercholesterolemia, smoking and overweight were more frequent in Eastern and South Eastern Europe (*WHO ERICA Project, 1998*). Austrian-Bulgarian comparable epidemiological study of CRF found that hypertension, elevated hematocrit and elevated lipoprotein were more frequent for the Bulgarian population while reduced physical activity was more frequent for the Austrian cohort. Bulgarian volunteers had more often increased cholesterol and decreased level of HDL while the ratio cholesterol/HDL was found with the same frequency in the two populations (*Lechner H, HadjievD 1998*).

Prospective cohort study of the risk factors for stroke conducted in Münster among 12, 866 men of age from 30 to 65 with duration of the observational phase of 7.2 years found that the relative risk (RR) for ischemic stroke was associated with high systolic arterial pressure - 2.99 (95% Cl, 0.85 to 10.49).

This risk was associated respectively with smoking of more than 20 cigarettes daily - 3.56 (95% Cl, 1.78 to 7.15) and with diabetes mellitus - 2.21 (95% Cl, 1.0 to 4.87) (*Berger K et al.1998*). Epidemiological study of CRF in the French population found that arterial hypertension was the most significant RF for ischemic stroke development. Smoking, diabetes mellitus, alcohol abuse and high fibrinogen levels were relatively associated with the risk for stroke while cholesterol showed relation to stroke development and opposite relation to cerebral hemorrhages. Besides, the relative risk for stroke significantly increased in patients who had suffered from transient ischemic attacks in the last 5

years compared to individuals who had not (*Zuber M, Mas JL 1992*).

Prospective cohort 20-years epidemiological study of 7, 052 men and 8, 354 women of age from 45 to 64 studied the role of the main risk factors for stroke - arterial hypertension, serum cholesterol, blood sugar, smoking, height, body mass index (BMI), preceding cardiovascular diseases and diabetes mellitus. It was found that the diastolic and systolic blood pressure, smoking, preceding cardiovascular diseases and diabetes mellitus were positively related stroke development while the forced respiratory volume per second and the height were negatively related to cerebrovascular incidents. Cholesterol did not show any relation to strokes while such was found when blood sugar was elevated. Smokers suffered more frequently from strokes than non-smokers while the relation between high BMI and strokes was not established for certain although individuals with higher BMI suffered more frequently from strokes (*Hart CL et al. 2000*). Population epidemiological studies in Asian regions confirm the role of the same risk factors for stroke. Studies conducted in Japan, Taiwan and Indonesia outlined the leading role of arterial hypertension, cardiovascular diseases, diabetes mellitus and smoking for stroke development (*Shimamoto T et al. 1996, Hu HH, Tzeng SS 1994; Vohra EA et al. 2000*). In case-control epidemiological study of CRF held in India by means of the logistic regression analysis was measured the role of five essential risk factors: hypertension (OR=1.9, 95% Cl, 1.5 to 2.5), total serum cholesterol (OR=2.3, 95% Cl, 1.4 to 4.9), use of anticoagulation and antiaggregation agents (OR=3.4, 95% Cl, 1.1 to 10.4), preceding transient ischemic attacks (OR=8.4, 95% Cl, 2.1 to 33.6), and alcohol consumption (OR=2.1, 95% Cl, 1.3 to 3.6). These RFs appeared to be significant for stroke manifestation (*Zodpey SP et al. 2000*). 5-years epidemiological study

of CRF in Thailand revealed that hypertension was the main risk factor for stroke while diabetes mellitus, smoking, alcohol consumption, hyperlipidemy and basic cardiovascular diseases were insignificant risk factors (*Viriyavejakul A et al. 1998*).

Cohort epidemiological study held in Australia for 98 months investigated the main risk factors for stroke. The created multivariate model gave the opportunity to find that the significant risk factors for stroke were the advanced age, male gender, preceding strokes, high blood pressure, atrial fibrillation, decreased HDL, reduced physical activity and depressions (*Simons LA et al. 1998*).

These as well as many other population-based epidemiological studies revealed the need of good knowledge and study of CRF in order to carry out effective primary and secondary stroke prophylaxis.

Some of the risk factors for strokes are well documented while the role of others is still not completely revealed. In that term, it was decided to divide CRF into two main groups - well and less well documented ones (*Stroke Council of the American Heart Association, 1997*).

II. CLASSIFICATION OF THE RF FOR CVD

A. Well documented risk factors
- ⇨ Arterial hypertension
- ⇨ Cardiovascular diseases (atrial fibrillation, ischemic heart disease, left ventricular hypertrophy - ECG, etc.)
- ⇨ Smoking
- ⇨ Asymptomatic carotid stenoses (ACS)
- ⇨ Diabetes mellitus
- ⇨ Transient ischemic attacks (TIA)
- ⇨ Other well documented risk factors

B. Less well documented risk factors
- ⇨ Dyslipidemy
- ⇨ Alcohol abuse
- ⇨ Reduced physical activity
- ⇨ Obesity
- ⇨ Elevated hematocrit and fibrinogen
- ⇨ Other less well documented risk factors

1. Well documented RF for CVD

1.1. Arterial hypertension

A big number of clinical and epidemiological studies showed that arterial hypertension is the basic risk factor for development of ischemic strokes and hemorrhages. According to the criteria of WHO arterial hypertension is a condition characterized by permanent elevation of systolic pressure above 160 mmHg and diastolic pressure above 95 mmHg. According to the same criteria blood pressure 140/90 mmHg is normal, and values between these grades are "borderline" *(Bakris G 1997)*. The analysis of the results from Framingham cohort study showed that arterial hypertension was the most important independent risk factor for development of atherothrombotic stroke. Morbidity of ischemic stroke elevated in a direct ratio with the elevation of blood pressure in all age groups *(Kannel WB 1996)*. Data from Framingham study showed also that the relative part of atherothrombotic stroke increased compared to the other types of strokes together with the increase of the severity of arterial hypertension from 38% to 61% in men and

from 25% to 64% in women. That meant in individuals with moderate to heavy hypertension prevailed atherothrombotic stroke but not parenchymatous cerebral hemorrhage *(Wolf P et al. 1986)*. The relative risk for

stroke in the age group from 35 to 64 was 11.2 in men and 13.6 in women and in the age group from 65 to 84 it was respectively 3.9 and 6.4 *(Wolf P et al. 1986)*. According to data from Framingham study the attributive risk for stroke in individuals with arterial hypertension varied depending on the age from 33.4% to 48.8% *(Wolf P 1993)*.

The project of WHO, ERICA, held in 17 European countries showed that arterial hypertension was most often in men from North Europe and in women from East and South Europe (*WHO ERICA Project, 1988*). In other wide epidemiological study of WHO, MONICA, held in 18 populations from 11 countries with total number of 2.9 million population was found hypertension incidence between 12 % and 42 % in men and between 10 % and 41 % in women. Arterial hypertension was mostly widespread in Finland and Germany and rarely in Denmark. It was found also a positive correlation between this risk factor and strokes for both genders but in men correlation was statistically insignificant (*Stegmeyer B et al. 1997*).

Based on the data from 12 epidemiological studies investigating 2379 cases of stroke, a relative risk of 5.43 (95% Cl, 4.62 to 6.39) associated with hypertension was found. The relative risk for hemorrhages was 5.44 (95% Cl, 3.99 to 7.40) and for ischemic strokes 5.25 (95% Cl, 3.95 to 6.98) (*He J et al. 1995*). Relative risk for arterial hypertension was high in other observations, too (*Lindenstrom E et al. 1995; Marand van de Mheen, PJ et al. 1998*). Relative risk for stroke for arterial hypertension varied according to the age. 6-year epidemiological study involving male population of the age from 45 to 81 revealed a significant increase in the thrombembolic strokes in patients with arterial hypertension compared to normotensive individuals with the increase of the age for both groups (*Curb JB et al. 1996*).

Arterial hypertension demonstrated different incidence depending on the type of stroke. Prospective epidemiological study among 248 stroke patients found that hypertension was the most frequent risk factor for intracerebral hemorrhages (83%), followed by the cases of lacunar infarction (82%), and patients with ischemic stroke (59%) (*Fonseca et al. 1996*).

Framingham study found that individuals with single systolic hypertension had higher stroke morbidity. The relative risk for all types of stroke in men with single systolic hypertension was 2.0 for the age group from 65 to 74 and 2.2 for the age group from 75 to 84 (*Wolf P et al. 1993*). 20-year epidemiological study held in Scotland revealed that systolic arterial pressure was more significant risk factor for males and diastolic one for females (*Carole L et al. 1999*). Single systolic hypertension turned to be a significant risk factor in Danish population. The relative risk for stroke was 2.30 (95% Cl, 1.6 to 5.3) for females and 2.7 (95% Cl, 1.8 to 4.3) for males and the population attributive risk was 30% (*Nielsen WB et al. 1996*). Prospective epidemiological study held in 23 clinical centers in England, Scotland and North Ireland involving 4, 801 volunteers showed that single systolic hypertension demonstrated significant correlation to macro- and microvascular disorders including strokes (*Adler AI et al. 2000*). Other observations conducted in different geographical regions also marked the leading role of single systolic hypertension for stroke occurrence (*Petrovich H et al. 1995; Davis BR et al. 1998*).

Data from nine huge prospective studies showed that there was a direct relation between the increase in the diastolic arterial pressure and morbidity of stroke and ischemic heart disease (*Mc Mahon et al. 1990*). Data from 12-year study of the mortality from stroke held in Oslo showed that the dominating role of increased diastolic pressure (*Haheim LL et al. 1995*). Epidemiological study of 4,736 individuals of age above 60 years found that on the background of increased diastolic pressure the relative risk for stroke was 1.14 (95% Cl, 1.05 to 1.22) and for coronary heart disease was 1.08 (95% Cl, 1.00 to 1.16) (*Somes CW et al. 1999*). Other wide study involving 40,551 individuals for a period of 11 years showed significant increase in the number of strokes in the Western and Eastern populations of the USA (*Ni Mhurchu et al. 1999*). Diastolic arterial pressure increasing in the interval of 90 and 110 mmHg significantly elevated the risk for strokes, coronary incidents and death but on the other hand, its medicinal treatment reduced this risk (*Hannekens CH 1998*).

The leading importance of the arterial hypertension as a risk factor for strokes suggested the need of medicinal and non-medicinal prophylaxis of this RF in the general strategy for treatment of cerebrovascular diseases.

1.2. Cardiovascular diseases

Cardiovascular diseases are the second of importance risk factor for stroke after arterial hypertension. Among them well documented RFs for stroke are atrial fibrillation, infectious endocarditis, mitral stenosis, acute
myocardial infarction and left ventricular hypertrophy (*Sacco RL et al. 1997*).

A significant number of RF have common responsibility for the occurrence of cardiovascular diseases and stroke: age, gender, social status, blood pressure, preceding heart disease, angina, myocardial infarction, diabetes, peripheral vascular disease, TIA'S, stroke, atrial fibrillation, fibrinogen, smoking and alcohol, high total cholesterol (*Quzilbash N 1998*). CVD usually go side by side with ST decrease and abnormal

T-waves as well as prominating U-wave and other polarization changes, and QT-interval elongation in the ECG (*Perron AD, Brady WL 2000*). Patients with cerebral ischemia have high mortality for the basic reason of myocardial infarction. Cohort multicenter randomized clinical study held among 3, 021 patients with TIA and strokes revealed that 189 died for heart reason. Multivariant analysis showed the following independent predisposing factors for cardiac pathology: age above 65 years, male gender, angina, and diabetes, frontal myocardial infarction, left ventricular hypertrophy and T-wave turn in the ECG. These data confirm the necessity of ECG investigations in patients with cerebral ischemia (*Pop GA et al. 1994*).

Cardiac risk factors for stroke were studied among 232 patients. It is found that the most common were ischemic heart disorders (48.2%), dysrhythmias (46.1%), stable angina (34.4%), ventricular weakness (13.4%), atrial fibrillation (12.5%), atrial flatter (12.5%), and experienced cardiac infarction (9.9%) (*Witczak et al. 1998*).

The most common mechanism for the occurrence of stroke was cardioembolic one followed by hemodynamic disorders and ateromatous changes in the vessels. The most common reason for embolism were dysrythmias and especially atrial fibrillation. The role of *foramen ovale*, experienced coronary bypass and aortic aterosclerosis was marked. About one third of the stroke patients had had asymptomatic disorders of the coronary circulation (*Sen S, Oppenheimer SM 1998*).

Another prospective population based study of 5 880 individuals of age 65 and older investigated cardiac RF for ischemic stroke. Population attributive risk increased with prior coronary diseases (13.1%), systolic arterial pressure = 140 mm Hg (12.8%), high level of C-reactive protein (9.7%), abnormal left ventricular function (4.8%) and atrial fibrillation (2.2%) (*Gottdiener JS et al. 2000*).

1.2.1. Atrial fibrillation

Atrial fibrillation (AF) is the most frequent cardiac arrhythmia. The Framingham study founded that its incidence increases with age and that it is two times more frequent among men compared to women. After 50 years of age the incidence of AF doubles for each further decade and reaches up to 10% in individuals 80-89 years of age (*Wolf PA et al. 1998*). AF is the most frequent and significant RF leading to cerebral infarction (*Albers GW 2000; Sen S, Oppenheimer SM 1998; Albers GW et al. 1997*).

Another prospective study of 1 197 individuals with acute stroke held in Denmark found 18% incidence of AF. This incidence increased with age in individuals with stroke: 2% for individuals of age 50; 15% for individuals of age 70; 28% for individuals of age 80; 40% for individuals of age 90. Multivariant analysis showed the relation between incidence of AF and: 10-year increase of age OR 2.0 (95% Cl, 1.6 to 2.6); ischemic heart diseases OR 3.4 (95% Cl, 2.4 to 4.8); previous stroke OR 1.8 (95% Cl, 1.2 to 2.0); and 10 mm Hg increase of systolic blood pressure OR 0.93 (95% Cl, 0.88 to 0.99).

There were no significant correlations to gender, diabetes, hypertension, TIA and "silent" strokes found on CT scans. There was a higher 50-day in-hospital mortality rate of patients with AF OR 1.7 (95% Cl, 1.2 to 2.5), (*Jorgensen HS et al. 1996*). 30-day stroke mortality rate in patients with AF (25%) was significantly higher compared to patients without AF (14%) OR 1.84 (95% Cl, 1.04 to 3.27), (*Lin HJ et al. 1996*).

A prospective comparable study investigated patients with ischemic stroke of age 65 or more who had paroxysmal atrial fibrillation (PAF), patients with paroxysmal atrial fibrillation of age under 65 and elderly people with chronic atrial fibrillation (CAF). Cases of all types of stroke in patients with PAF in the age group of 65 years (4.8%) were significantly more rarely than those in the CAF group and more frequently compared to the young patients group with stroke incidence of 2.5% per year. Cerebral embolism had incidence of 2.7% in the age group of 65 and older and was significantly more rarely than those in the CAF group (5.1%) and higher than those found in younger patients (1.3%) annually (*Nakajiama K, Ichinose M 1996*).

A clinical and pathological study of 136 patients with stroke and non-rheumatic atrial fibrillation (NAF) receiving anticoagulant therapy was conducted. Strokes (with certain symptoms present) were found in 82 patients (63%) with NAF and they were significantly more frequent than those of control group - 55 (23.8%). More frequent in the NAF group were also cardioembolic, atherotrombotic, and lacunar strokes compared to those in the control group. Incidence of stroke mortality was also significantly higher in the NAF group than in the control group. Pathomorphologic study of individuals over 70 years of age showed that srokes

(with certain symptoms present) NAF was 2.5 times more frequent than in the control group without NAF (*Yamanouchi H et al. 1997*).

Yearly risk of NAF was about 4.5% but analysis of five controlled epidemiological studies showed that this risk decreased to 1.4% in patients with anticoagulant and antiaggregant therapy including *Warfarin* and *Acetysal* (*Koefoed BG et al. 1996*).

NAF increased the risk of ischemic stroke especially in individuals with left ventricular hypertrophy, left ventricular insufficiency and left atrial enlargement (*Yoshida M et al.1996*).

In patients with atrial fibrillation were often observed "silent" strokes (*Ezekowitz MD et al.1995*).

A population-based cohort study of 2 635 patients of age 75 and older investigated the mortality in patients with stroke and AF. The relative mortality risk on the 28th day was 1.25 (95% Cl, 1.4 to 1.5), and at the end of the first year it was 1.4 (95% Cl, 1.18 to 1.67). Cox-proportional hazardous model showed that the stroke mortality risk in patients with AF was significantly higher than in the patients without AF – 1.24 (95% Cl, 1.10 to 1.39), (*Kaarisalo MM et al.1997*). Another study showed that in patients with AF the relative risk was 1.56 of non-embolic strokes, 5.80 of embolic ones, and 1.31 of death (*Yuan Z et al.1998*).

Population attributive risk of stroke in patients with chronic non-rheumatoid atrial fibrillation increased in ☒ direct ratio with age. In the age group of 50-59, it was 1.5% and reached about 30% for the age group of 80-89 (*Wolf PA et al. 1987*).

1.2.2. Ischemic heart disease (IHD)

Ischemic heart disease (IHD) is not only a source for cardiocerebral embolism but also concomitant disease in patients with cerebrovascular disease due to the similar risk factors. In the presence of IHD, the risk of atherothrombotic stroke was two times higher (*Wolf PA et al. 1987*). Patients with stroke in the past were of higher risk of myocardial infarction (*Wang TD et al. 1997*), and the presence of coronary heart disease might worsen the prognosis of cerebrovascular disease. A great number of patients with ischemic impairment of cerebral circulation (from 20% to 40%) have IHD (*Nishino N et al.* 1993; *Thomas M et al.* 1999). A prospective epidemiological study among 14 371 middle-aged men from Finland showed that inherited coronary diseases among women had significant effect on stroke incidence while in men such a relation was not established (*Jousilahti P et al.* 1997).

An investigation of incidence and severity of asymptotic coronary diseases in patients with different types of stroke was made. 65 patients with TIA and ischemic stroke without any symptoms of coronary heart disease were evaluated with stress test to find the reasons for the cerebral ischemia. The frequency of abnormal stress tests was 50% in patients with large vessel disease while in patients with other reasons for cerebral ischemia it was 23%. Patients with penetrating arteries disease or cryptogenic stroke had significantly lower incidence of asymptotic coronary diseases than those with large vessel disease. Large vessel disease, smoking, and left ventricular hypertrophy may lead to TIA and stroke, that
in crease the risk of asymptotic coronary diseases (*Chimowitz MI et al.* 1997).

Ultrasound investigation of individuals with carotid artery atherosclerosis and atherosclerosis of peripheral arteries as well as quantitive angiography of patients with coronary atherosclerosis were made to evaluate the level of vascular impairment. The results showed significant correlation between the atherosclerotic changes found by ultrasonography of the carotid bulb, and the marrow parts of the coronary arteries. Another significant correlation was found between the atherosclerosis of peripheral vessels and the diameter of the stenotic parts of the coronary segment (*Hulthe J et al.* 1997).

Patients with carotid stenosis had higher incidence of asymptotic heart diseases. 444 men with carotid endarterectomy due to asymptotic carotid stenosis were evaluated. Clinical examination and ECG investigation were made to determine the presence of pectoral angina and myocardial infarction. During the study 86 patients (43%) with coronary disease and 81 patients (33%) without disease passed ischemic heart attack. The factors related to heart attacks in patients without coronary disease were diabetes OR 2.14 (95% Cl, 1.15 to 3.97), intracranial occlusive disease OR 2.13 (95% Cl, 1.13 to 4.02), and peripheral vascular diseases OR 2.04 (95% Cl, 1.14 to 3.36). In conclusion, individuals with carotid stenosis without coronary disease suffered rarer from heart attacks than those who had had such. On the other hand, patients with carotid stenosis without coronary disease but with intracranial occlusive disease, diabetes, and peripheral vascular diseases had risk similar to that of individuals who had had heart attacks (*Chimowitz MI et al. 1994*).

Another study of a Spanish population found that "silent" strokes could be observed in patients with coronary disease (*Modredo – Pardo PJ et al. 1998*). These investigations confirmed the relation between IHD and ischemic impairments of the cerebral circulation. The relative risk of ischemic stroke in patients with IHD was 2.6 (95% Cl, 1.13 to 6.01), (*Nishino N et al. 1993*), while the attributive risk of stroke in patients with IHD was 9% (*Thomas M et al. 1999*).

The risk of stroke in patients with coronary disease was reduced significantly under effective antiaggregant treatment (*Mahaffey KW et al. 1999*). That fact confirmed the need of right prophylaxis of IHD as a part of the entire strategy for stroke treatment.

1.2.3. Left ventricular hypertrophy

Left ventricular hypertrophy is well documented stroke risk factor (*Sacco R et al. 1997*). Framingham study showed that ECG proved left ventricular hypertrophy increased four times the risk of stroke (*Wolf P et al. 1987*).

A prospective epidemiological study of 5 201 men and women 65 years of age and older and duration of 3.3 years found that left ventricular hypertrophy increased significantly the risk of stroke, together with the age, impaired glucose tolerance, high systolic arterial pressure, carotid stenoses, and atrial fibrillation (*Menolio TA et al. 1996*). Another population-based 8-year study of 447 men and 783 women 67 years of age and older investigated the influence of left ventricular hypertrophy on stroke incidence. Stroke risk in individuals with left ventricular hypertrophy was defined by proportional hazardous regression multivariant analysis after evaluation of the following factors: age, gender, systolic

arterial pressure, antihypertensive treatment, diabetes, smoking, and serum lipid levels. The relative risk of ischemic stroke in individuals with left ventricular hypertrophy was 1.45 (95% Cl, 1.17 to 1.80) (*Bikkina M et al.* 1994).

On the other hand, the hemispherical strokes seemed to be a significantly related reason to the continuous and persistent impairment of the autonomous cardiac regulation in abnormal changes of the heart sizes (*Korpeleinen JT et al.* 1996). A number of surveys revealed the relationship between the increased left ventricle size and the risk of stroke and lethal outcome. A population-based trial investigating patients age 50 and older for a period of eight years established dilated left atrium. In that case 4% of men and 4.2% of women have had stroke and 21.6% of men and 15.7% of women died. Considering gender-specific Cox - a proportional hazardous model after taking into account the age, presence of hypertension, diabetes, atrial fibrillation, smoking, proven by ECG left ventricular hypertrophy, heart failure, and myocardial infarction, it was shown that each increase by 10 mm in the left atrial sizes revealed a relative risk of stroke in men 2.4 (95% Cl, 1.6 to 3.7) and in women 1.4 (95% Cl, 1.0 to 2.1). The relative risk of death was 1.3 (95% Cl, 1.0 to 1.5) in men and 1.4 (95% Cl, 1.1 to 1.7) in women (*Benjamin EJ et al.* 1995). Acute left ventricular dysfunction and thrombosis in the left ventricle could be observed in cerebral hemorrhage by ultrasound investigation (*Misumi I et al.* 1997).

By ECG left ventricular hypertrophy was associated with the increased mortality of cardiovascular diseases in hypertensive conditions (*Frimm CD et al.* 1999).

Measurement of left ventricular mass and systolic function was done by means of *Cardiothoracic ratio* x 100. The increase of this parameter led to an increase of the relative risk of stroke in men 1.17 (95% Cl, 1.03 to 1.32) and in women 1.07 (95% Cl, 0.95 to 1.19) (*Carole L et al.* 1999).

The prognostic value of a new ECG method for left ventricular hypertrophy diagnostics in essential hypertension was investigated (*Perugia score*) compared to the standard ECG methods in 1, 717 hypertensive patients of mean age 52.

Multivariant analysis showed an independent relation between left ventricular hypertrophy and the risk of cardiovascular diseases - *Hazard Ratio* (HR 2.04,

95% Cl, 1.5 to 2.8). Population attributive risk of cardiovascular disease accounted to 15.68% for all the cases *(Verdecchia P et al.1998)*.

1.3. Smoking

Smoking belongs to the well documented and treatable RF of cerebrovascular disease. Nicotine and the rest of the wasted products from tobacco burning impair vessel endothelium and favors atherogenesis.

Ultrasonographic investigation held in Sweden population of healthy individuals of age 35-60 found that continuous smoking for a long time led to considerable atheromatous changes in the carotid arteries. Side by side the cholesterol level elevated *(Bolinder G et al.1997)*. Other prospective survey showed that smoking had a key role for high grade carotid stenoses development. In that survey, the effect of smoking on American and German population was compared. High grade carotid stenoses were found in 14% of the investigated from the American population and in 21% from the German one. After taking into consideration the impact of the rest of the RFs as age, gender, hypertension, diabetes, hypercholesterolemia, and ethnic belonging, the multivariate logistic regression analysis gave the opportunity to define the chances ratio for stenoses occurrence. In both nationalities smoking showed an

independent relation to the carotid stenoses - for the American population OR 1.5 (95% Cl, 1.1 to 2.0) and for the German one OR 3.9 (95% Cl, 2.4 to 6.3). Severity of the carotid stenoses was associated in a direct ratio with the increase in the number of smoked cigarettes *(Mast H et al.1998)*.

Besides, smoking worsened the blood rheologic properties by enhancing the platelet activity and increasing fibrinogen plasma concentrations and plasminogen activator PAI-1 concentrations *(Zidovetzki et al.1999)*.

The role of smoking for stroke occurrence was assessed by Framingham cohort study. It was found that the relative risk of stroke in smokers was 1.5 to 2.9 times higher than those in non-smokers. This risk increased with the increase in the number of smoked cigarettes. When consuming more than 40 cigarettes daily the risk was twice as higher compared to smokers consuming up to 10 cigarettes daily. After quitting smoking for 2 years, the risk of stroke considerably decreased *(Wolf PA et al.1988)*.

The risk of stroke with fatal outcome was investigated in Swedish population of 16, 209 smokers of age 40-49 for a period of 18 years. The results from the proportional hazardous regression analysis after considering the impact of other RFs as age, diastolic arterial pressure, and blood glucose concentration revealed that combined

smoking of cigarettes and pipe suggested relative risk 6.1 (95% Cl, 3.0 to 12.5) and consuming only cigarettes the risk is 4.1 (95% Cl, 2.3 to 7.4).

Smoking of cigarettes increased the risk of stroke by 3.5 times *(Haheim LL et al.1996)*.

Analysis of the results from 32 epidemiological studies showed that smoking carried a relative risk of stroke in

smokers equal to 1.51 compared to non-smokers and this risk was higher in women *(Shinton R et al.1996)*.

By means of longitudinal epidemiological study held for a period of 12.5 years among 7, 735 men of age 40 to 59 the risk of fatal and non-fatal stroke was investigated. It was found that the relative risk of stroke in smokers (RR 3.7 95% Cl, 2.0 to 6.9) was four times bigger than those in non-smokers. Quitting smoking by consumers of up to 20 cigarettes daily led to significant decrease in the risk of stroke while in consumers of more than 40 cigarettes daily the cessation of this harmful habit had poorly decreased the risk of stroke *(Wannamethee SG et al.1995)*.

A study of the American Oncological Society held among 1.2 million people for a period of six years had calculated an attributive risk of death as a result of pulmonary carcinoma, chronic obstructive pulmonary disease, coronary heart diseases, and stroke. This risk exceeded 19% *(Malarcher AM 2000)*.

In some cases smoking favors the occurrence of "silent" strokes. It is found also a significant reduction of HDL in smokers compared to non-smokers *(Yamashita K et al. 1996)*.

Apart from smoking being a risk factor of stroke, it is the reason for considerable economic losses related to the treatment of the diseases caused by it. The investigations conducted in Germany and England found an abundant financial expenditures for the treatment of caused by smoking socially significant diseases, i.e. myocardial infarction, stroke, atherosclerotic vascular diseases, pulmonary carcinoma, etc. *(Ruff KL et al. 2000; Naido, B et al. 2000).*

These data shows the need of conducting an active prophylaxis directed in smoking cessation which will

have not only favorable health impact but also will lead to significant saving of financial sources for other treatments.

1.4. Asymptomatic carotid stenoses

It is known that atheromatous process is the most common reason for inner carotid arteries stenosis or occlusion. Stenoses and ulcerated atheromatous plaques are localized usually at the bifurcation region and not rarely they are multiple. Atherosclerotic plaques constrict the vascular lumen and lead to reduction of the regional cerebral blood flow and if they ulcerate, microembolization of the cerebral arteries occurs. Carotid stenoses, even the most severe ones, might remain without clinical manifestation, i.e. asymptomatic carotid stenoses (ACS). It is found that ACS refers to the well documented and treatable RF of CVD *(Sacco RL et al.1997).*

The first population-based study of ACS distribution by means of Doppler sonography was held by *Ricci, S* et al. (1991). It found that 5% of the population of age above 49 had proven homodynamic stenoses above 50%.

By means of numerous other population-based epidemiological studies conducted via various ultrasound techniques was found that high grade carotid stenoses are present in 4% to 8% of adult population *(Mannami Tefal.1997; OLeary et al 1992; Pujia A et al. 1992).*

ACS are far more usual among patients with cardiovascular diseases. In peripheral angiopathies carotid stenoses more than 50% are found in 25% to 35% of the investigated individuals *(Cheng SW et al. 1999; House AK et al. 1999).*

Longitudinal population-based epidemiological studies revealed that the risk of ischemic cerebral circuit disorders increased with the escalation of ACS grade. *J.W.Norris* et al. (1991) showed via Doppler sonography that the annual risk of ischemic stroke in individuals with ACS above 75% or less was 1.3%. In these cases the combined risk of myocardial ischemia and vascular death was significantly higher, i.e. 9.9% annually. Severe stenoses above 75% had combined risk of TIA'S and stroke of 10.5% annually. And 75% of the ischemic vascular lesions develop at the site of the stenotic artery.

Other multicenter longitudinal population-based epidemiological study using ultrasound methods revealed that severity of ACS was the most important factor which allowed to make a prognosis of the occurrence of neurological and other complications. Annual morbidity of ischemic stroke, homolateral to ACS, was above 1.4% when it is 80% or less. However, when ACS was above 80% the annual morbidity of ischemic cerebral circulatory disorders increased triple *(Mackey AE et al. 1997).*

Other observation conducted by means of ultrasonographic techniques found that 5-years risk of fatal and non-fatal stroke, homolateral to ACS, was 5%. Individuals with ACS above 70% experienced ten times bigger risk compared to low grade stenoses *(Longstreth H et al. 1998).*

The mentioned results showed that stenoses which were hemodynamically significant were not only indicative for diffuse atherosclerosis but also preceded ischemic cerebral circulatory disorders in the stenotic artery pool. The incidence of these disorders increased with the escalation of stenosis grade. It was found that the incidence of "silent" strokes visualized by MRI (Magnetic Resonance Imaging) increased significantly in the presence of severe carotid stenoses and ulcerated
atheromatous plaques. These infarctions were more frequent at the site of carotid impairment *(Houdaku H et al. 1994).*

Some randomized studies found that ACS was a local factor in the pathogenesis of ischemic cerebral circulatory disorders *(Hobson RW et al. 1993).*

Population-based epidemiological studies revealed that elevated serum LDL, high systolic arterial pressure and smoking were the main RFs for ACS occurrence *(Sharret AR et al. 1999).* In men these correlated to the age, systolic arterial pressure, impaired glucose tolerance, smoking, serum cholesterol and decreased HDL. In women considerable relationships between them and the age, systolic arterial pressure, impaired glucose tolerance and serum cholesterol were established *(Mannami T et al. 1999).*

Crucial interest arose from the studies dedicated to progression and regression of ACS as well as to their determining factors. In men of age 65.5 dynamic sonographic investigations for a period of 28 months revealed annual risk for stenosis progression of 9.3%. It is found that the relative progression risk depends on the stenosis grade in the inner and outer homolateral carotid arteries and on the stenosis grade in the contralateral

inner carotid artery as well as on the elevation of systolic pressure above 160 mmHg *(Muluc SC et al. 1999).*

In some cases, ACS underwent a certain regression. Catamnesic angiographic investigation for a period of 22 months found that high grade stenoses diminished in 10% of the patients *(Chaturvedi S et al. 1994).*

The mentioned data provided the arguments to assume that ACS were not only a sign of diffuse atherosclerosis but also a local factor with important role in the

pathogenesis of cerebral ischemia. Frequently, ACS combined with other CRFs like arterial hypertension, cardiovascular diseases, diabetes mellitus, hyperlipidemias, etc. which enhanced their unfavorable role in the pathogenesis of strokes. Discovering ACS nessecitated medicinal treatment and in some cases, operative treatment as well. Medicinal therapy was directed to management of the basic risk diseases and operative treatment usually was performed in the cases of severe stenoses involving from 75% to 99% of the lumen of the carotid artery. Thus, an effective primary prophylaxis not only of ischemic cerebral circulatory disorders but also of myocardial infarction might be done.

1.5. Diabetes mellitus

Diabetes mellitus is an important factor in the cerebrovascular disease development. It causes endothelial proliferation and impaired function of plasmic membranes of the minor blood vessels. Diabetes mellitus provides conditions for development of atherosclerotic changes in the vascular walls and worsens rheological properties of the blood and thus, increases the risk of thrombotic and embolic changes *(Santos-Lasaosa S et al. 2000).* It leads to various and persistent complications in almost all the organs and systems in the organism like nephropathies (29%), neuropathies of the peripheral nerves (25.1%), hypertension (23%), obesity (21.3%), coronary heart diseases (21%), retinopathies (15%), hypercholesterolemia (11%), stroke (5.6%), etc. *(Weerasuriya N et al.* 1998). A particularly great bunch of these cardiovascular risk factors was observed in diabetes mellitus type II *(Kaukua J et al.* 2001). Usually strokes developed in the phase of renal insufficiency (34%) *(Schleifer T et al.* 1998).

Framingham study demonstrated that the risk of ischemic stroke was twice higher in patients with diabetes mellitus compared to healthy individuals.

Diabetes mellitus was found in 7, 735 (2.1%) individuals in a prospective cohort study held in Scotland among 366, 849 people registered by their general practitioners. The presence of diabetes mellitus type II resulted in increase of the risk of myocardial infarction and stroke and both types of diabetes, I and II, caused increased risk of endocrine and metabolic disorders or renal insufficiency *(Donnan PT et al.* 2000).

Longitudinal epidemiological study of cohort of 408, 000 individuals demonstrated that morbidity of CVD in diabetic patients was from 23‰ to 32.8‰ while in individuals without diabetes it was from 2.4‰ to 3.3‰. Consistent with the age, the relative risk for diabetic men was 3.37 (95% Cl, 3.53 to 3.88) and for women it was 4.35 (95% Cl, 4.37 to 4.76) *(Currie CJ et al.* 1997). Other population-based study revealed that diabetic patients with stroke were with 3.2 years younger than investigated individuals without diabetes. According to Jorgensen H et al. (1994) cerebral hemorrhages were 6 times more often in diabetic patients while Mankovsky BN et al. (1996) reported that diabetes mellitus was a RF only for ischemic stroke.

The risk for ischemic stroke development increased due to continuous course of diabetes and in the presence of some of its complications. Prospective trials dedicated to diabetes type I and II found abnormal increase of the urinary albumin excretion, hypertension, smoking, and poor metabolic control *(Parving HH* 1999).

The relationship between hyperglycemia in individuals without diabetes and stroke in some cases was significant and in others was not proven yet. Metaanalysis of three longitudinal studies held among 98,

783 individuals for a period of 12.4 years showed that the relative risk of cardiovascular diseases was 1.58 (95% Cl, 1.19 to 2.10) at blood glucose level of 7.8 mmol/l compared to blood glucose level of 4.2 mmol/l *(Countincho M et al. 1999)*. Impaired glucose tolerance was not significantly related to ischemic strokes while proven diabetes mellitus had a serious correlation to development of stroke (OR, 1.6, 95% Cl, 1.0 to 2.6) and myocardial infarction (OR, 1.9, 95% Cl, 1.3 to 2.8) *(Qureshi AJ et al. 1999)*. Except from this, plasma glucose concentration above 8 mmol/l, measured post experienced acute stroke incident, worsened the final outcome prognosis *(Weir CJ et al. 1997)*.

High glucose concentration is a risk factor for death in individuals who are not diabetics. Longitudinal epidemiological studies found that high glucose concentration in healthy individuals of middle age was a significant risk factor for death due to stroke and myocardial infarction *(Balkau B et al. 1998; Orencia AJ et al. 1998; Slowik A et al. 1998)*.

Diabetes mellitus is a powerful RF for death due to stroke for both gender. Prospective trial involving 8, 077
men and 8, 572 women for a period of 16.4 years found a relative risk for death due to stroke of 1.7 and 3.7 for women *(Tuomilehto J et al. 1996)*. Other case-control study with 15 years duration conducted among diabetic patients type II found that cardiovascular mortality was significantly higher in patients compared to the control group *(Niscanen L et al. 1999)*.

Considerable part of diabetic complications are associated with the progression of atherosclerotic changes. High resolution properties of current ultrasonographic investigations give the opportunity to make a non-invasive assessment of the atherosclerotic changes in blood vessels. Case-control study held among 244 healthy individuals and 240 insulin-dependent patients investigated atheromatous changes in the common carotid artery. Multiple lineal regression analysis showed considerable impact of diabetes mellitus, increased total cholesterol and tryglicerides, decreased HDL and older age for development of atheromatous changes in carotid arteries *(El-Barghouti N et al. 1997)*. Combined influence of these RFs for development of atherosclerotic changes in carotid arteries were found in other similar observations, too *(Teno S et al. 2000)*.

The role of diabetes mellitus as an independent and treatable RF of CVD imposes the need of its treatment and prophylaxis in time yet before the complications development.

1.6. Transient ischemic attacks

Transient ischemic attacks (TIA'S) are acute cerebral circulatory disorders that are accompanied by focal neurological symptoms caused by insufficiency of the cerebral blood flow. Clinical manifestations continue usually from 2 to 15 minutes and totally fade away no later than 24 hours. TIA'S tend to recur and usually end with the development of cerebral infarctions for a different period of time.

According to Framingham study data they compose 15% of the cerebrovascular incidents *(Wolf PA.* 1990).

Risk factors of TIA'S and cerebral infarctions are analogous.

TIA'S refer to the well documented and treatable RFs of stroke *(Sacco RL et al.* 1997). The relationship between clinical symptoms of TIA'S and cerebral infarctions, and supposed RFs for their occurrence was established via logistic regression method. The relationship between the manifestation of these symptoms and diabetes mellitus , smoking, hypertension, poor education, high lipoprotein levels, hemostatic factor VIII and *von Willebrand* factor was statistically significant. Apart from this, carotid intimal medial thickness above 1.17 mm for men and above 0.85 for women defined by Doppler sonography is

associated with twice as higher risk of TIA'S and cerebral infarctions occurrence *(Chambless LE et al.* 1996). Other similar survey found that hypertension and preceding TIA'S on one hand and atrial fibrillation on the other hand, correlated to the occurrence of lacunar infarctions *(Toni D et al.* 1995).

It was pointed out that annual risk of stroke in TIA'S patients is 3.7% *(Easton JD* 1997).

By means of case-control method was found that the risk of stroke among patients with TIA'S was 5.5% (95% Cl, 3.7 to 8.5) *(Whisnamt JP* 1997). Prospective case-control study found the relationship between TIA'S and other RFs of stroke, and progression of cardiovascular disorders. It was determined that 21% of the patients with TIA'S had developed other vascular incidents and

8.1% had died of cardiovascular diseases. In the control group 18% had developed other incidents and 5.4% had died of cardiovascular diseases. Patients with TIA'S had 2.3 times higher risk of stroke development compared to controls *(Mortel KF et al. 1996)*.

In other investigation held by case-control method, the multiple logistic regression analysis provided the opportunity to measure ORs for each risk factor. The final model added to the age and date of the stroke incident included TIA'S, hypertension, smoking, atrial fibrillation, ischemic heart disease, mitral valve diseases and diabetes mellitus *(Whisnamt JP et al. 1996)*.

Some cluster studies are present aiming to assess the absolute and relative risk for stroke recurrence for a long period of time. Repeated strokes usually are associated with the presence of preceding TIA'S, atrial fibrillation, male gender, hypertension, alcohol consumption, smoking, diabetes mellitus, ischemic heart disease and increased serum levels of cholesterol and hematocrit *(Jorgensen HS et al. 1997)*.

TIA'S outcome prognosis depends on many and various factors. Prospective trial on mortality rate among individuals with TIA'S found that it was much more higher compared to patients with mild stroke. Patients with TIA'S had more often intermittent claudication and more often died from myocardial infarction compared to the group with mild stroke *(Falke P et al. 1994)*. Other surveys were dedicated to TIA'S and strokes outcome prognosis in young individuals. It was found that the severity of the first stroke was the only prognostic sign of disability *(Ferro JM et al. 1994)*. Mean annual rates of occurrence of new strokes, myocardial infarctions and lethal outcome were higher in patients with combined atherothrombotic and cardioembolic pathogenesis compared to the rest of the patients. Male gender and age above 35, early experienced stroke and cardiovascular diseases were independent RFs which were worsening the outcome *(Marini C et al. 1999)*. Apart from this, it is

found that epileptiformic seizures in first 48 hours of the stroke development and TIA'S were independent prognostic factor for hospital mortality *(Arboix A et al. 1997)*.

Patients with TIA'S who had hemodynamically significant carotid stenoses and especially of the type above 80% of the carotid lumen were extremely endangered of strokes *(Ellis MR et al. 1992)*.

Early diagnostics and secondary medicinal and operative prophylaxis of TIA'S provide the opportunity to reduce morbidity and mortality due to cerebral and myocardial infarctions.

1.7. Other well documented risk factors

To this group refer some blood diseases like sickle cell anemia and some disorders of aminoacid metabolism like increased plasma homocystein concentrations which is a risk factor for carotid atherosclerosis and ischemic stroke.

Growing older is associated with an increase in the risk for stroke especially after the age of 55 and stroke morbidity for both genders escalates almost twice through every ten years. It is also found that stroke predisposition for some individuals is great and among Afro-Americans strokes are more often compared to Caucasian. Gender, age, family predisposition, and ethnic belonging as well as geographic location refer to the well documented but non-treatable and impossible to prophylact risk factors of stroke.

2. LESS WELL DOCUMENTED RISK FACTORS

2.1 Dyslipidemies

It is found that dyslipidemy was important and treatable RF for ischemic heart disease. Considerable number of
studies were recently dedicated to clarifying of its role in the occurrence of ischemic cerebral circulatory disorders.

Serum lipids and lipoproteins consist of cholesterol, triglycerides, low density lipoproteins (*LDL*), very low density lipoproteins (*VLDL*), and high density lipoproteins (*HDL*).

WHO ERICA Project found that hypercholesterolemia was most common in women from the investigated Northern and Eastern Europe populations. For men it was most popular in Northern Europe. The incidence of hypercholesterolemia for both genders was lowest among the investigated population from Southern Europe in whose nutrition the relative part of saturated fatty acids was the smallest (*The WHO ERICA Project 1998*).

Great geographic differences were found in distribution of hypercholesterolemia during result analysis of WHO MONICA Project. Increased plasma cholesterol concentrations were found in 3% to 51% of the investigated men and in 4% to 44% of the investigated women (*Stegmeyer B et al.* 1997a).

Data about hyperlipidemia as a RF of stroke were gathered from a number of longitudinal epidemiological studies and from investigations using case-control method.

It was shown via earlier studies that total cholesterol, HDL, and LDL were RFs for TIA'S and strokes with mild neurological insufficiency (*Qizibash N et al.* 1991). Based on the data from 10 prospective studies, it was measured that the relative risk for stroke at present hypercholesterolemia was 1.31(*Qizibash N et al.* 1992).

A newer prospective study found that total cholesterol is a RF for ischemic stroke only when its plasma concentrations exceeded 8 mmol/l. The risk of ischemic stroke increased also with the elevations of triglycerides but decreased with the elevation of plasma HDL (*Lindenstrom E et al.* 1994). It was pointed out that the relative risk of ischemic stroke for dyslipidemia varied between 1 and 2 (*Sacco RL et al.* 1999).

On the contrary to these data via analysis from 45 prospective cohort studies was indicated that there was no relation between the level of plasma cholesterol and stroke. These studies, however, did not specify the type of stroke and for that reason the positive correlation between cholesterol and stroke could be masked by its negative correlation to cerebral hemorrhage (*Prospective Studies Collaboration* 1995).

Despite that hypercholesterolemia was not accounted to the well documented RFs of stroke, current studies had convincingly proven the existence of relation between plasma lipids and risk of ischemic stroke (*Sacco RL et al.* 1997a).

A number of epidemiological studies using ultrasound techniques indicated that there was relationship between hypercholesterolemia and carotid stenoses development (*Wilson PW et al.* 1997).

The difference in the data about the role of dyslipidemia as a RF of ischemic stroke was possibly due to the fact that in most of the population-based studies the heterogeneity of strokes was not taken into account. On one hand, it was proven that dyslipidemiae were

RFs for atherothrombotic stroke and on the other hand, it was known that low concentrations of plasma cholesterol combined with arterial hypertension was a RF for
cerebral hemorrhage (*Girond M et al.* 1995; *Jacobs DR* 1994).

2.2 Alcohol abuse

A number of epidemiological studies showed that alcohol consumption was related to the risk of ischemic and hemorrhagic strokes.

The role of chronic consumption of moderate alcohol amounts (less than 60 g ethanol per 24 hours) in ischemic stroke genesis is still under discussion. Two basic cohort studies revealed that even the moderate alcohol consumption increased the risk of hemorrhagic strokes (*Camargo CA* 1996). Other study found that consumption of 1 g to 20 g alcohol daily the previous week led to significant decrease of morbidity of ischemic stroke and intracerebral hemorrhages (*Jamrozik K et al.* 1994).

Framingham study showed that the relationship between alcohol consumption and stroke occurrence was possibly present only in men and alcohol abuse usually was accompanied by arterial hypertension and smoking. This was confirmed in other trials, too (*Starr J M et al.* 1996; *Known SU et al.* 2000).

The relative risk for stroke and cerebral hemorrhages was measured via controlled study involving four group of patients which were separated according to the amount of the consumed alcohol: 1 g to 90 g; 100 g to 390 g; 400 g and above this amount per week. The individual risk counted to 1.0 : 0.6 : 0.7 : 2.4 for strokes in men and women (*Gill GS et al.* 1991).

Currently held 13.5-years prospective epidemiological study among 7, 735 men of middle age who consumed more than 60 g ethanol daily revealed a relative risk for
stroke of 1.9 (95% Cl, 1.0 to 3.5) for the first 8 years. After taking into account the impact of systolic arterial pressure, however, the risk was reduced to 1.5 (95% Cl, 0.8 to 2.7). The relative risk for stroke in low and moderate consumers of alcohol was lower than for those
who drank great amounts and did not differ from the risk of individuals who drank irregularly. However, this did not mean that low

and moderate amounts of alcohol had protective effect against strokes (*Wannamethee SG et al. 1996*).

Population attributive risk for stroke in chronic alcohol abuse was 4.7% (*Gorelick PB 1995*).

ORs were calculated via multivariate logistic regression analysis for different amounts of alcohol abuse as RF for stroke. Regular considerable alcohol abuse but not its cessation was an independent RF for stroke; the relative risk was 1.82 (95% Cl, 1.8 to 3.5). Alcohol consumption in amounts of 150 g to 300 g and above 300 g weekly preceded stroke occurrence and significantly increased the risk for cardioembolic and cryptogenic stroke; the relative risk was respectively 3.61 (95% Cl, 1.67 to 7.79) and 3.74 (95% Cl, 1.61 to 8.73). Consumption of more than 40 g alcohol in the previous 24 hours increased the risk for cardiogenic cerebral embolism especially among individuals with marked atherosclerotic changes in the main arteries; the relative risk was 7.68 (95% Cl, 1.82 to 32.3). Mild consumption of alcohol did not increase the risk for stroke (*Hillbom M et al. 1999*). Other similar survey found that the risk for stroke significantly increased when consuming above 60 g daily but in that case the intake of this dose in the previous 24 hours was not a risk factor (*You RX et al. 1997*).

The dominating part of epidemiological studies provides the arguments to assume that chronic alcohol abuse is a
RF for strokes. However, considering strokes, these data are still controversial especially when low and moderate
amounts of alcohol are consumed.

2.3 Reduced physical activity

Although limited in their size, studies held in the last years revealed that moderate physical activity decreased significantly the risk for stroke while the reduced one predisposed to its development.

Case-control prospective epidemiological studies were held in which reduced physical activity was indicated as a RF for stroke together with hypertension, atrial fibrillation, carotid stenoses, diabetes mellitus, smoking and TIA'S (*Elking MS, Sacco RL 1998*). Other longitudinal cohort study with mean duration of 11.6 years investigated the risk for stroke when physical activity was reduced. This reduction was graded as low, moderate and high. After taking into account other RFs as age, smoking, diabetes mellitus, cardiovascular disease, education, and systolic arterial pressure, *BMI*, serum cholesterol and hemoglobin concentration, the relative risk for stroke was measured. The relative risk was highest for women, i.e. 1.82 (95% Cl, 1.10 to 3.02) but tendency to increase was observed in men, too. The results gave the arguments to the authors to suggest that moderate physical activity might lead to reduction of stroke incidence for both gender (*Gillum RF et al. 1996*). Prospective cohort study continuing for 9.5 years found that the relative risk for stroke was respectively 1.0 for low, 0.6 for moderate and 0.3 for high physical activity. However, very intense physical activity did not have protective properties while moderate one led to reduction of the risk for stroke and myocardial infarction in men

with or without ischemic heart disease (*Wannamethee G, Shaper AG. 1992*). Other longitudinal cohort study continuing for 15 years found that the relative risk for heart attacks and strokes as well as mortality significantly increased with smoking and $BMI > 26$ kg/m^2 and statistically significantly decreased with

moderate physical activity. On the other hand, moderate immobilization led to increase of the relative risk for cardiac and cerebral infarction (*Wannamethee SG et al. 1998*).

Case-control study indicated that physical activity during spare time turned to be protective in terms ischemic stroke occurrence. This effect was accounted for all age groups, for both genders and for all ethnic groups included in the study (*Sacco RT et al. 1998*).

2.4 Obesity

Overweight refers to the less well documented and treatable RFs for ischemic stroke. The degree of obesity is quantitatively assessed by body mass index (*BMI*) that is accepted as pathologic in cases when its values exceed 27.3 kg/m^2 0 kg/m^2.

WHO ERICA Project investigating risk factors of ischemic heart disease found that mean population *BMI* is higher in South-Eastern than in North-Western Europe and the differences were more marked in women (*The WHO ERICA Project 1998a*).

Overweight is usually combined with other risk factors like CVD. A highly risk population for stroke development including 550, 000 residents in 22 regions were investigated. The risk for stroke was positively associated with the increase of age, blood pressure, blood sugar, cholesterol and *BMI*, and these RFs were detected in 71.43% of the patients with stroke (*Guo Z et al. 1996*).

Case-control study revealed that the combination of smoking and reduced physical activity was present in 62% of the patients with stroke and the combination of obesity and smoking in 72% of the patients. On the other hand, not a single case of stroke was registered with the
lack of smoking, obesity and hypodynamic lifestyle (*Shintom R 1997*).

It is assumed that abdominal obesity might be more dangerous for stroke than general obesity. The relationship between *BMI* and abdominal obesity in ratio (waist-hip) with stroke incidence was studied. Compared to the men with lowest *BMI*, the men with highest *BMI* had adapted to the age relative risk for stroke of 1.29 (95% Cl, 0.73 to 2.27). To the opposite, the adapted to the age relative risk for extreme values of the waist-hip ratio was 2.33 (95% Cl, 1.25 to 4.37). A small correlation to the waist measurement was found and men with the biggest measured waist showed a relative risk of 1.52. The results showed that the abdominal obesity defined the risk for stroke and not the *BMI*.

Studies dedicated to obesity as an independent RF for stroke were poor and controversial. It was pointed out that obesity was associated with arterial hypertension, high levels of blood sugar and serum lipids which were independent RFs for stroke (*Sacco RL 1997a*).

Despite the controversial data about the role of the obesity as an independent RF fro stroke, its impact might be assumed proven. This fact imposed normalization of the overweight to be included in the complex prophylaxis programs for limiting cerebrovascular and cardiovascular diseases.

2.5. Increased hematocrit and fibrinogen

Impaired rheologic properties of blood introduce a risk for ischemic strokes by causing reduction of the cerebral blood flow and favoring atherogenesis and thrombogenesis. The basic rheologic factors which decrease the cerebral blood flow with their increase are hematocrit and fibrinogen. Blood viscosity is significantly higher in acute and chronic cerebral infarctions and plasma viscosity increases also in ACS, TIA'S and vascular dementia (*Coul BM et al. 1991; Fisher M, Meiselman K 1991*).

Epidemiological studies revealed that increased above 0.45 hematocrit was a RF for ischemic strokes development. Hematocrit is most significantly associated with total serum proteins, total cholesterol, triglycerides, systolic and diastolic blood pressure and heart rate (*Wannamethee G, Shaper AG 1994*). Smoking has a specific impact on the rheologic properties of blood. It is found that smoking led to increase of hematocrit and plasma fibrinogen and therefore, results in increased viscosity (*Ernst E 1995*).

Prospective cohort study was held within 9.5 years investigating the risk for stroke at hematocrit values =51%. After taking into account the impact of the other RFs like age, social belonging, smoking, *BMI*, physical activity, preceding heart disease, diabetes mellitus and systolic pressure, the relative risk for stroke reached 2.5 (95% Cl, 1.2 to 5.0). However, the increased hematocrit was associated with higher incidence of strokes only in men with hypertension. These data indicated that hematocrit increase is an independent RF for ischemic stroke and the risk increases with the increase of blood pressure (*Wannamethee G et al. 1994*). Besides, it was found that blood viscosity and hematocrit increased in men with atherosclerosis of the inner carotid artery (*Carralo C et al. 1998*).

Except hematocrit, increased fibrinogen also worsens the rheologic properties of blood mainly by inducing reversible platelet aggregation. Fibrinogen also participates in the formation of atherosclerotic plaques by stimulating proliferation and migration of smooth muscle cells in the vascular wall. A number of epidemiological studies revealed that increased fibrinogen was an independent RF for ischemic stroke development. Factors influencing the level of plasma fibrinogen are mainly age, smoking, gender and genetic predisposition. Dynamic investigation of population of patients with strokes indicated that levels of fibrinogen were three times higher in men with B - beta 448 genotype three months after the beginning of the vascular incident (*Carter AM et al. 1997*).

In patients with acute ischemic stroke the arterial hypertension affected the participation of fibrinogen molecules in red blood cells' interrelations (*Kowal PA 1996*). Coagulation disorders were studied in patients with lacunar cortical stroke. Levels of fibrinogen, *von Willebrand* factor, prothrombin factors 1 and 2, anti-thrombin III, protein C and protein S were measured. Statistically significant increase in coagulation activity was found in the gr up of patients with cortical stroke compared to healthy individuals. Besides, a considerable increase in the level of fibrinogen and *von Willebrand* factor was observed in these patients compared to the group of patients with lacunar stroke (*Giroud M et al. 1998*).

These two parameters were significantly increased in patients with "quiet" multiple lacunar strokes compared to the non-lacunar ones (*Kario K et al. 1996*).

Studies demonstrated that the increased hematocrit and fibrinogen were independent RFs for ischemic strokes. They are treated as less well documented but treatable factors (*Sacco RL et al. 1997*).

2.6. Other less well documented risk factors

They include some medications, irrational nutrition, migraine, hypercoagulability, some infections and social-economic factors.

Oral contraceptives have unfavorable effect over the hemostasis by causing hypercoagulability and fatty profile disorders. Prospective cohort study conducted among women aged from 25 to 39 who had used oral contraceptives found a relative risk for stroke of 2.9 (95% Cl, 1.3 to 6.7) (*Mant J et al. 1998*).

The impact of migraine on stroke occurrence is still under discussion due to the fact that it is usually accompanied by other vascular risk factors like smoking, oral contraceptives, hypertension, etc.

It is known that abuse with salty, sweet and fatty food favors the development of asymptomatic ischemic cerebral circulatory disorders but the relationship between the impaired nutrition and strokes has not been established yet.

The role of some other less well documented RFs for stroke like social-economic status, emotional stress and geographic life conditions is still a subject of investigation.

III. Descriptive and analytical studies of RFs for CVD in our country

The presence of high and increasing morbidity, contagiosity and mortality from CVD is observed by all Bulgarian investigators studying these group of disease in our country - Z. Bogdanov, G. Nastev, 1972, D. Hadgjiev, R. Rashev, 1978, G. Molhov et al. 1980, T. Cholakov et al. 1989, L. Coneva-Pencheva, 1983, 1988, N. Golemanov, 1986, 1991 (*Merdganov Ch,* 1995).

Basic RFs for CVD were studied. The role of smoking was studied by Hadgjipetrova E (1980), Manchev I (1989), and Shotekov P (1992) as a risk factor for strokes (*Merdganov Ch,* 1995a).

A lot of Bulgarian authors confirmed the importance of diabetes mellitus as a serious RF for cardiovascular diseases - T. Staikov et al. 1987, F. Grigorov et al. 1992, A. Penev 1984, K. Pavlov 1989 (*Merdganov Ch,* 1995b).

Other surveys in our country were associated with studying of less well documented RFs for CVD whose incidence in the total population of the investigated individuals was 8.1% and among patients with ischemic heart disease it was 91.5%. It was also found that every second Bulgarian (age 15-80) was overweight between 25 kg/m^2 and 30 k/m^2. These data revealed that obesity was the most popular among treatable RFs for CVD (*Merdganov Ch,* 1995c).

Epidemiological studies on alcohol abuse were held by T. Stankushev (1991) and N. Beshkov (1991). They indicated that alcohol abuse was found in 28.8% of the residents of cities and in 32.2% of the residents of villages (*Merdganov Ch,* 1995d).

According to Bulgarian authors - P. Slunchev and P. Angelova (1992) -hypodynamic lifestyle started in childhood and enhanced in older age groups (*Merdganov Ch,* 1995e).

P.Shotekov (1992) investigating pathology of extracranial cerebral arteries pointed out that the basic RFs for CVD, i.e. arterial hypertension, cardiovascular diseases, diabetes mellitus, smoking and increased alcohol consumption, usually combined with each other in development of inner carotid thrombosis in young men.

The problem of RFs for socially significant diseases in our country was most detailed discussed by Ch. Merdganov (1995f). The author followed and analyzed this issue in the last few decades.

A current Austrian-Bulgarian population-based epidemiological study of the cerebrovascular factors found that arterial hypertension was more frequent in Bulgarian population while cardiovascular diseases, smoking and diabetes mellitus had almost the same incidence in both populations. Hypercholesterolemia was more frequent in Bulgarian population while hypodynamic lifestyle was more common among Austrian volunteers (*Lechner K, Hadjiev D* 1998).

TIA'S refer to the basic RFs for CVD. Longitudinal epidemiological studies found contagiosity of 4, 040 of 100, 000 population of the age 40-59 (*Hadjiev D et al.* 1989).

Epidemiological studies held so far in our country investigating CRFs were to a great extent insufficient and one-sided, and gave a partial idea of the essence of a certain problem. They were not longitudinal but one-moment trials and therefore, they did not give the opportunity to follow the incidence dynamics of the different well and less well documented RFs for CVD. The incidence and structure of the numerous treatable CRFs were not investigated and followed dynamically. The RFs for ischemic stroke by case-control method were not investigated, too.

Due to the different social-economical conditions in our country by the time these old studies took place, there were no contemporary epidemiological, electrophysiological and biochemical investigation methods used for the studied populations and therefore, no sufficient data by its volume and content was obtained concerning these problems.

All these reasons suggest the necessity of longitudinal epidemiological studies for CRFs with respect to the great distribution of CVD in our country and also to improvement of the primary prophylaxis of these socially significant diseases.

IV. Problems under discussion

A number of longitudinal population-based epidemiological studies revealed that some RFs (arterial hypertension, cardiovascular diseases, diabetes mellitus,
smoking, hyperlipidemias, increased hematocrit and fibrinogen) could be treated while others (age, gender, family predisposition, ethnic belonging) could not be affected. Geographic differences in morbidity and mortality of strokes can be to some extent explained with the different distribution of RFs like arterial hypertension, smoking, hyperlipidemias, etc. On the other hand, the differences in distribution incidences of CRFs might be due to the differences in the clinical, laboratory and instrumental bunch of methods used for their identification. An unified screening method for identifying of CRFs is still missing and important role for this have also the different financial resources of the different countries and regions.

A considerable amount of clinical-epidemiological trials indicated that arterial hypertension was the basic RF for CVD. Its treatment reduced the risk for stroke from 30% to 42%.

Cardiovascular diseases (, atrial fibrillation, left ventricle hypertrophy and heart failure) are independent RFs for stroke. Ischemic heart disease is the most important among them.

Diabetes mellitus increases the risk for stroke but rarely it is an independent RF. It usually combines with arterial hypertension.

Smoking has been also referred to the well documented and treatable RFs for CVD. Like diabetes, this RF rarely acts independently. Smoking usually shows relation to the occurrence and progression of atheromatous changes of blood vessels. It often combines with alcohol abuse, arterial hypertension, cardiovascular diseases, etc.

The role of symptomatic carotid stenoses for the development of ischemic cerebral circulatory disorders is known for ages. Studies dedicated to ACS are insufficient and in some aspects their importance is under discussion. A number of one-moment population-based epidemiological studies using ultrasound techniques revealed that hemodynamically significant ACS were found in 4% to 8% of the adult population and the incidence of hemodynamically insignificant ACS varied between 28% and 54%. According to some surveys the 5-years risk for stroke homolateral to the ACS was 5%. If stenoses were severe (involving above 70% of the arterial lumen), the risk was ten times higher than those for the low grade stenoses. The relationship between ACS and diabetes mellitus, reduced HDL, systolic arterial pressure and cardiovascular diseases was revealed. The relationship between ACS and smoking was confirmed by some authors and disputed by others. Following the dynamics of ACS it was observed that they progressed with the increase of the age but sometimes they might also regress. The incidence of ischemic stroke occurrence cited by the various studies was also different which confirmed the need of conducting longitudinal studies to investigate this problem.

Big differences were also observed in the incidence of less well documented RFs for stroke represented by the various studies. These were found in WHO ERICA and MONICA Projects. The latter project revealed great geographic differences in hypercholesterolemia distribution which varied from 3% to 51% for the investigated men and from 4% to 44% for the investigated women. Based on the data from the conducted prospective cohort studies was found that cholesterol increased the relative risk for stroke but on the contrary to these data, other observations indicated that there was no relation between plasma cholesterol level and strokes. However, the relation between hypercholesterolemia and carotid atheromatosis was found for sure. Population-based studies held by case-control method reported that HDL had statistically significant protective properties against stroke.

Prevalent part of epidemiological studies gives the arguments to assume that chronic alcohol abuse is a RF for strokes. However, data considering cerebral infarctions is still controversial especially drinking of small and moderate amounts of alcohol which are not proven to increase the risk for stroke and some authors even suggest that these amounts exert protective action.

Hypodynamic lifestyle and obesity do not act as independent RFs for stroke and usually combine with smoking, hypertension, cardiovascular diseases and diabetes mellitus.

A number of epidemiological studies are dedicated to distribution of the different RFs for CVD but few of them focus on the combinations of RFs and their prognostic importance. Well and less well documented

RFs for ischemic stroke usually combine. Taking into consideration the RFs which cannot be affected (age, male gender, race, ethnic belonging and family predisposition), CRFs most usually are combined. The distribution of combinations of well and less well documented RFs for ischemic stroke has not been a subject of special population-based epidemiological study. Therefore, for the sake of primary and secondary prophylaxis of stroke it is of special importance to identify the individuals with multiple CRFs who can be treated in time. With respect to all these, there is a need of conducting longitudinal epidemiological studies by means of which to identify and assess both the single and multiple CRFs in order to prevent the development of different types of CVD.

V. PERSONAL INVESTIGATIONS

Based on the conclusions made from literature overview of RFs for CVD and taking into consideration some of the unsolved problems of epidemiology and prophylaxis of these conditions, we have conducted two-phase population-based epidemiological study among 500 healthy individuals (200 men and 300 women) at age 50-79 for defining the incidence of RFs in our country as well as their natural dynamics and outlining some issues for their prophylaxis.

All individuals were investigated by means of instrumentation provided by Austrian-Bulgarian study of CRF.

5.1. Results from population-based epidemiological study of Cerebrovascular risk factors

Well documented risk factors for cerebrovascular disease

5.1.1. Arterial hypertension

5.1.1.1. Merdganov Ch (1995) made analysis of the conducted so far epidemiological studies in our country investigating arterial hypertension and emphasized on their positive features and respective methodic disadvantages. He summarized the results from the conducted screening trials of arterial hypertension and indicated that approximately 1 million from the investigated 1.4 millions population of age 15 to 84 had blood pressure values of 160/95 mmHg. The author emphasized that arterial hypertension was one of the basic risk factors for the development of cardiovascular and cerebrovascular diseases.

Another study of us held by S. Torbova (1994) among the population in the capital found the presence of arterial hypertension in 42% of women and 34% of men at age 55 to 64 and after age of 65 this incidence was respectively 66% to 26%.

Austrian-Bulgarian comparative population-based epidemiological study of cerebrovascular risk factors revealed that arterial hypertension in the age group of 49 to 74 was found in 61.2% of the investigated individuals from Sofia and in 40.2% of the Austrian population (Lechner H, Hadjiev D 1998a).

The distribution of the investigated individuals by gender and age is represented in **Table 1**.

Table 1

GENDER	AGE 50-59	* 60-79	TOTAL
Men	96	104	200
Women	158	142	300
Total	254	246	500

*Note: The second group of investigated individuals is distributed in the age interval of 60-79 years because the individuals above 60 years of age are only 24. The bigger number of the women included in our study is due to the fact that the number of men above 50 years of age the investigated region is less that those of the women (17, 705 men and 20, 011 women). Besides, it is well known that women often participate in such trials.

Arterial hypertension is more often found in the age group of 60-79 years where it is respectively 49.3% for the women and 46.2% for the men and the differences between the different groups are not statistically significant. The smallest is the incidence of this RF among men of age

50-59 (38.5%). During the first investigation systolic hypertension is found in 199 of the investigated individuals (39.8%). This RF is usually found in age group of 60-79 years where it is respectively 47.9% for the women and 42.3% for the men. Increased diastolic pressure is also found with higher incidence among individuals of older age group. However, there is a certain impression that compared to the increased total arterial pressure and systolic hypertension, diastolic hypertension is more common among men (43.3%) than among women (41.5%).

With respect to studying the dynamics of arterial hypertension distribution, a repeated screening in the same population and by the same methods was conducted in two years and nine months. 418 individuals have come to the repeated examination which accounts to 83.6% of the investigated volunteers at the first examination. Seven individuals died for this period: 4 of cardiovascular diseases and 3 of malignancies. The rest 71 individuals did not come although they were invited several times. At the second examination a tendency to increase in the incidence of arterial hypertension in women for both age groups was recognized as well as for men aged 60-79, while in men from the age interval of 50-59 years this incidence was relatively small.

The increase of the incidence of arterial hypertension is statistically significant and associated with the increase in the age for all the investigated groups ($p < 0.05$). Compared to the first observation, the second one was characterized with increase in the number of hypertensive patients with the total of 43 individuals while only in 7 of the investigated volunteers this parameter had been normalized.

Dynamics of the changes in the arterial hypertension rates for both age-and-gender groups at the first and second investigation is represented in **Figure 1**.

Figure 1

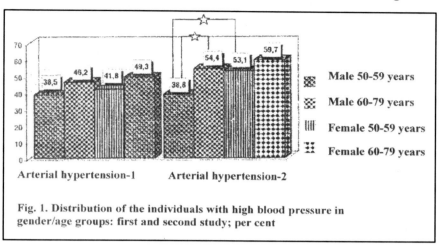

Fig. 1. Distribution of the individuals with high blood pressure in gender/age groups: first and second study; per cent

It was found that there was a statistically significant increase in the incidence of arterial hypertension at the second trial compared to the first one among men ($p < 0.001$) and among women ($p < 0.0001$).

At the second investigation the systolic hypertension was once again most common among the examined individuals of age 60-79.

There was a statistically significant increase in the incidence of systolic hypertension along with the increase of the age of the investigated population ($p < 0.05$). The increase of the number of patients with systolic hypertension was statistically significantly higher among men of age 60-79 compared to younger men ($p < 0.05$). Besides, this increased systolic pressure

was more often among women of age 50-59 compared to the men of the same age ($p < 0.05$).

The dynamic follow up of the number of individuals with systolic hypertension found that there was increase in the incidence at the second investigation compared to the

first one. And while in men of age 50-59 this increase turned to be insignificant, in men of the age interval 60-79 ($p < 0.05$) and in women from the first ($p < 0.001$) and the second ($p < 0.001$) age groups this increase was statistically significant **(Figure 2)**.

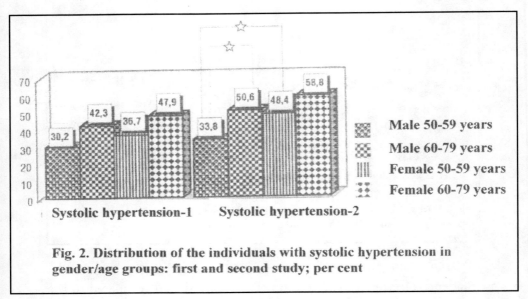

Fig. 2. Distribution of the individuals with systolic hypertension in gender/age groups: first and second study; per cent

Diastolic hypertension at the second investigation was most frequent among women of age 60-79 (55.5%) and 50-59 (50.8%) followed by the one reported in older men (49.4%).

Significantly higher incidence of this RF was found among women of age group 50-59 compared to the men of the same age ($p < 0.0001$). Diastolic hypertension was statistically significantly higher also among older men compared to the younger men ($p < 0.05$).

At the second observation there was a significant increase in the number of individuals with diastolic hypertension, i.e. 42 individuals were with newly found hypertension while only in 7 volunteers the values of this parameter were normalized. At the same time diastolic hypertension showed statistically significant increase in its incidence with the increase in the age of the investigated individuals ($p < 0.01$). Diastolic hypertension had been statistically significantly increased in men of the age 60-79 and in both groups of women (respectively $p < 0.01$ and $p < 0.0001$) (**Figure 3**).

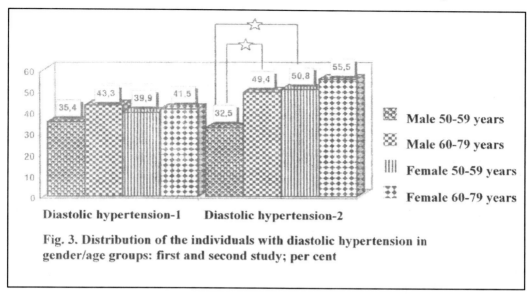

Fig. 3. **Distribution of the individuals with diastolic hypertension in gender/age groups: first and second study; per cent**

It is seen from the figure there is an increase in the incidence of diastolic hypertension in all of the investigated individuals at the second trial.

The current population-based epidemiological study of CRF clearly outlined the wide distribution of arterial hypertension whose incidence increased with the age. At the first trial the differences in the rates of this RF were not statistically significant while at the second one hypertension was more frequent among women of the age interval 50-59 compared to the men of the same age. At the second trial systolic and diastolic arterial hypertension were more frequent among women of age 50-59 and among men of age 60-79 compared to the younger men. Compared to the results from the Austrian-Bulgarian epidemiological study, the incidence of arterial hypertension among the investigated population was similar to that of the Austrian population, i.e. 40.2% (Lechner H, Hadjiev 1998b) but it was bigger than the reported one by the WHO ERICA Project. The difference is the most expressed compared to the Western European countries in which the arterial hypertension in the age group of 40-59 years was found 23.8% for men and 18.7% for women (the WHO ERICA Project, 1988). Despite almost the same incidence of systolic and diastolic hypertension (Schrader J et al.; Sesso HD et al. 2000), a number of investigations revealed that systolic hypertension had prevalence as a risk factor for cerebral circulatory disorders (Medical Research Council 1985, Menotti A et al. 1998, Staessen JA et al. 1999). Special high risk carried the critical increase in the arterial pressure (Otsuka K et al. 1997).

Prevalent role of the arterial hypertension as a RF for stroke was confirmed also by administration of antihypertensive therapy leading to moderate decrease in the values of systolic and diastolic arterial pressure. This decrease resulted in significant reduction of clinical cases with stroke (Ambrosioni E, Baaccelli S 1998; Suter PM et al. 1998; Rigand AS et al. 2000). The results from the conducted 14 randomized studies indicated a reduction of morbidity by 42% as a result of the carried out 5-year antihypertensive therapy (Collins R et al. 1990).

Ischemic cerebral circulatory disorders in arterial hypertension develop as a result of arteriosclerosis and functional disorders of the cerebral hemodynamics. Hypertension is recognized as a leading RF for stroke but its role in the occurrence of various types of CVD is not the same. Population-based epidemiological study held among 1057 hypertensive patients with stroke diagnosed on the basis of Lausanne Stroke Registry via methods of the logistic regression analysis found that arterial hypertension was not always a leading factor for cerebral hemorrhages, and cerebral and lacunar infarctions had occurred more often in the presence of older age, smoking, diabetes mellitus, preceding TIA'S, family predisposition, hypercholesterolemia, etc. (Lestro - Henriques I et al. 1996). Cerebral hemodynamics was disturbed also as a result of enhancement of the atherogenesis and the higher incidence of carotid stenoses in older patients with arterial hypertension (Franklin SS et al. 1997).

Besides, the arterial hypertension led to impairment of the cognitive function and development of vascular dementia (Guo Z et al. 1998; Kilander L et al. 1998).

The leading role of the arterial hypertension as a risk factor for cerebrovascular disease imposes administration of antihypertensive medicaments in time and also non-medicinal treatments in the prophylaxis and therapy of strokes.

5.1.2. Diseases of the cardiovascular system

The role of diseases of the cardiovascular system and especially of some of them like atrial fibrillation, infectious endocarditis, fresh myocardial infarction and mitral stenosis in occurrence of TIA'S and ischemic stroke is outlined by a number of Bulgarian authors (Merdganov Ch 1995, Shipkovenska E 2001). So far, there are single population-based studies dedicated most of all to the distribution of ischemic heart disease (Vulkov J 1996). It was currently held a longitudinal population-based epidemiological study of the cerebrovascular RFs which showed the importance of cardiovascular diseases for the occurrence of ischemic cerebral circulatory disorders (Manchev I 1999).

5.1.2.1. Atrial fibrillation

At the first study atrial fibrillation was most common in the subgroup of individuals of age 60-79 where its incidence was 8.0% for the women and 3.4% for the men. This RF was not found in men of the age 50-59.

At the second study held after a period of two years, again atrial fibrillation was more common among the investigated individuals of age 60-79 - 8.8% for the men and 6.1% for the women.

5.1.2.2. Ischemic heart disease

At the first study ischemic heart disease was more common in the group of men aged 60-79 (6.6%) and 50-59 (4.5%) and it was not found in older women.

The incidence of ischemic heart disease at the control observation had significantly increased for all age groups and it was highest among men of age 50-59 (43.8%).

5.1.2.3. Left ventricular hypertrophy

At the first study left ventricular hypertrophy (at the ECG) was most common in men of age subgroup 60-79 (6.8%) and was comparatively rare in the rest of the population of healthy individuals.

Two years after the background investigation the incidence of left ventricular hypertrophy did not show significant changes in the investigated by our staff population.

In that case left ventricular hypertrophy had been also most common among men of the older age group (8.8%).

Figure 4 reveals the distribution of individuals with cardiovascular disease by gender and age for both studies.

Figure 4

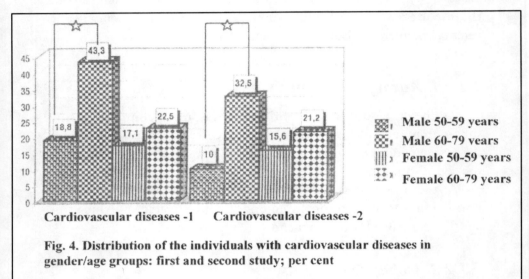

Fig. 4. Distribution of the individuals with cardiovascular diseases in gender/age groups: first and second study; per cent

At the first study cardiovascular diseases in men were significantly more frequent in the age subgroup 60-79 compared to the subgroup between 50-59, i.e. 43.3% and respectively 18.8% ($p < 0.0001$). The difference in the distribution of cardiovascular diseases was also significant between men and women of the age subgroup 60-79, i.e. 43.3% and respectively 22.5% ($p < 0.001$).

At the second study cardiovascular diseases prevailed again among men of the age 60-79 - 32.5% compared to those of 50-59 - 10.5% ($p < 0.001$). They were significantly more frequent in older men and women ($p < 0.001$).

The dynamic follow up of the incidence of cardiovascular diseases did not show significant change at the second study compared to the background study with the exception of ischemic heart disease which increased.

The incidence of cardiovascular diseases discovered among the investigated by our staff individuals varied between 18.8% and 43.3% at the first study and between 10.5% and 32.5% at the second one and was close to the reported in the Austrian-Bulgarian study for both populations (Lechner H, Hadgjiev D 1998c). The fact that with the increase of the age the incidence of cardiovascular diseases for both genders also increased deserved to be mentioned but this increase was statistically significant only for men. The larger distribution of cardiovascular diseases was notable among men of the age group 60-79 compared to the women of the same age. Data from the Framingham study indicated that with the increase of the age the role of chronic non-rheumatic atrial fibrillation as a risk factor for ischemic stroke increased (Wolf PA 1993).

The importance of atrial fibrillation for the genesis of ischemic strokes was marked by many other authors (Shively BK et al. 1996; Yuan Z et al. 1998). The relationship between the degree of carotid stenoses, smoking and atrial fibrillation was found, too (Ruivo A et al. 1996). Atrial fibrillation was found with various incidence in the different geographic regions and among different ethnic groups (Truelsen T et al. 1994; Hajat C et al. 2001). It was recommended that anticoagulant and antihypertensive prophylaxis of atrial fibrillation was done with respect to reduction of the risk for stroke (Albers GW et al. 1997; The SPAF III 1998).

Longitudinal study in Rochester and other studies revealed that the increased morbidity of strokes at least partially can defined by the increase in the relative part

of patients with ischemic heart disease and acute myocardial infarction (Brown R et al. 1996; Kubota K et al. 1997; Mooe T et al. 1997).

Left ventricular hypertrophy found by the ECG investigation also carried a risk for development of ischemic stroke and showed relation to the progression of carotid atherosclerosis (Vaitkus PT et al. 1995; Okin PM et al. 1996; Chlumsky J, Charvat J 2000).

Frequently, the impact of cardiac risk factors in the development of ischemic strokes was combined with other risk factors like for example, atrial fibrillation, arterial hypertension and ischemic heart disease with smoking, diabetes mellitus, dyslipidemias, etc. (Jedrzeiowska H et al. 1996; Bilora F et al. 1996; Cooper R et al. 2000).

It was pointed out that heart failure, atrial fibrillation and cardioembolic stroke were more frequent in older patients while strokes due to atherosclerotic changes of the magistral arteries were found usually among younger patients (Pohjasvaara T et al. 1997).

Cardiovascular diseases can be positively affected by systemic prophylaxis and treatment. In order to reduce the risk for ischemic stroke it is necessary that patients with atrial fibrillation, ischemic heart disease, left ventricular hypertrophy and other more rare diseases to be followed up by constant observation and to be included in time in appropriate prophylactic programs.

5.1.3. Smoking

The epidemiological studies held in our country dedicated to the distribution of smoking revealed that this RF was found in more than 40% of the population at the age above 20 years. Approximately 3 million Bulgarians are suffering from the negative effect of smoking. The

risk for stroke is more than three times higher among smokers compared to non-smokers and the highest is the relative risk in younger age groups (Hadgipetrova E 1980). Significantly increased the number of smokers under 20 years of age in the latest years (Tomov I 1992).

The more longer the duration and higher the intensity of smoking was, the bigger was the atherogenic risk (Doichinov A 1978).

Mortality of smokers followed for a period of 15 years was higher compared to individuals who did not smoke (Merdganov Ch 1995).

Another Bulgarian authors - D. Hadgjiev, I. Manchev, P. Mungov, O. Tachev, L. Tconeva-Pencheva, P. Shotekov, V. Petrunyashev - also confirmed the role of smoking as a RF for CVD (Merdganov Ch 1995).

The differences in the distribution of smoking by gender and age were big. For both genders it was more often in the age group of 50-59 ($p < 0.0001$). The incidence of this well documented RF was higher among men (p < 0.0001). Smoking showed a clear tendency to decrease with the increase of the age especially among women aged 60-79 (4.9%).

At the second study a decrease in the incidence of smoking in men for both subgroups was observed where it was respectively 36.3% and 21.5% while in women these rates almost did not change.

At the second study smoking also was found more frequent among the investigated individuals aged 50-59. Its incidence was statistically significantly higher than the reported among men and women of the older age group (p < 0.0001). In that case also smoking was more frequent among men rather than among women (p < 0.01).

The result analysis showed a significant decrease of smoking rate at the second study compared to the first one totally for the whole population (p < 0.0001). Statistically significant decrease of the incidence of this risk factor was found in the subgroup of men at the second observation compared to the first one (p < 0.0001). The dynamics of these changes is represented in **Figure 5**.

Figure 5

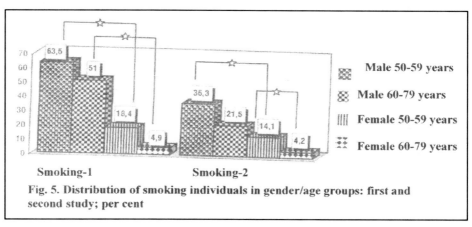

Fig. 5. Distribution of smoking individuals in gender/age groups: first and second study; per cent

Smoking for both age groups was significantly more frequent for men and its incidence decreased with the age. Smoking in the investigated by our staff population had significantly higher distribution compared to the two population studied in the Austrian-Bulgarian study (Lechner H, Hadgjiev D 1998). It is known that smoking refers to the well documented RFs for stroke (Sacco RL et al. 1997). Recently, it was demonstrated that for adults with single systolic hypertension, smoking and diabetes

mellitus were important risk factors for lacunar stroke (Davis BR et al. 1998).

Another study marked the relation of smoking to the occurrence of "quiet" strokes. Quitting smoking resulted in decreasing of this type of stroke (Howard BR et al. 1998). Besides, a direct ratio between the number of smoked cigarettes per day and the incidence of strokes was found. Men smoking 25 and more cigarettes daily had twice as higher mortality of stroke than those found for non-smokers (Carole L et al. 1996).

Smoking cessation led to favorable results in men and women from all age groups. Compared to smokers who did not overcome this bad habit, individuals who had quitted smoking demonstrated lower morbidity rate of cardiovascular diseases and mortality of cardiovascular and cerebrovascular diseases. Excessive coronary risk decreased almost half time from the first year after smoking cessation while a significant decrease in the incidence of cerebrovascular diseases was found in five years. These data indicated the need of elimination of this risk factor in the general strategy of prophylaxis of cerebrovascular diseases.

5.1.4. Asymptomatic carotid stenoses

The role of asymptomatic carotid stenoses (ACS) for the occurrence of ischemic cerebral circulatory disorders was revealed in a number of epidemiological studies but there are only few studies held in our country. For the first time P.

Shotekov (1986) carried out trials dedicated to the pathology of carotid arteries in our country and for this purpose he used confirmed international criteria for assessment the degree of stenoses. The problem is

discussed in details in the later on studies of this investigator (Shotekov P 1998, 1998a).

Population-based epidemiological study of hemodynamically significant asymptomatic carotid stenoses (Manchev I, Mineva P 1998) and their importance was emphasized in the occurrence of cerebral ischemia (Hadgjiev D et al. 1999). Population-based epidemiological study dedicated to the multiple cerebrovascular risk factors found that hemodynamically significant ACS participated in approximately 1/5 of the combinations of multiple mixed risk factor (Hadgjiev D et al. 1999a).

The incidence of ACS under 50% was highest among women of age 60-79 (61.3%) followed by this of the younger one (56.3%). For both gendersit was 54.6% (95% Cl, 50.2 – 54.6).

Stenoses above 60% were also most frequent for women in both groups (respectively 10.6% and 5.7%). For both genders it was 6.4% (95% Cl, 4.49 – 9.01).

The differences in the incidence of hemodynamically insignificant and hemodynamically significant ACS between the investigated men and women as well as between two age groups were not essential.

At the second study hemodynamically insignificant ACS were again more frequent among women of both age groups and the incidence for the whole population accounted to 57.9% (95% Cl, 53.2 – 62.6). It is found a statistically significant increase of the incidence of low grade ACS above 60 years of age for both genders.

At the second study hemodynamically significant ACS were found in 7.4% (95% Cl, 7.3 – 7.5) of the investigated individuals and again they were more frequent among women.

In 15.6% of the individuals with hemodynamically significant ACS a progression of the stenosis was found. In 9.4% of the investigated individuals from the age group 60-79 the hemodynamically significant stenosis of the inner carotid arteries was bilateral.

For the two years period of follow up in 12.5% of the investigated individuals with stenosis under 50%, a regression of the carotid stenosis was found.

No statistically significant differences between the maximum systolic and diastolic rates of the progressing and regressing stenoses at the first and second study were found.

For low grade ACS during the two years period of study in 9 (3.3%) of the investigated individuals, ischemic cerebral circulatory disorders occurred: TIA'S in 5 (1.8%) and stroke in 4 (1.5%) volunteers. For two years period of follow up of the participants in the study in 3 (9.4%) of them with hemodynamically significant ACS ischemic cerebral circulatory disorders (ICCD) were registered in the stenotic homolateral carotid pool: TIA'S in 6.25% and ischemic strokes in 3.13%.

In the cases without carotid stenoses for the two years period of follow up TIA'S in the carotid pool was observed in one volunteer (0.5%) from the age group 60-79 and myocardial infarction in one man (1.05%) from the age group 50-59.

The dynamic follow up of the ACS incidence by gender and age at the first and second observation showed an increase of the number of individuals with hemodynamically insignificant and hemodynamically significant ACS with the increase of the age and especially after 60 years of age (**Figure 6**).

Figure 6

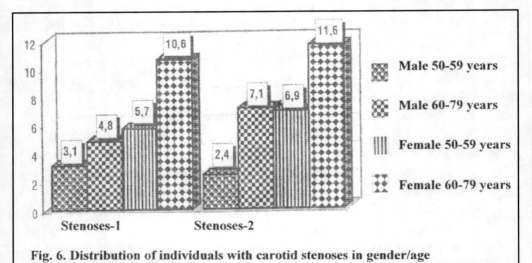

Fig. 6. **Distribution of individuals with carotid stenoses in gender/age groups: first and second study; per cent**

The cases of ischemic cerebral circulatory disorders in the carotid pool (78%) prevailed to those in the vertebro-basillar system (22%). Two (2.1%) of the men with low grade ACS in the age group of 60-79 suffered from myocardial infarction and in one of them it was combined with cerebral infarction.

Statistically significantly higher rates of ischemic cerebral circulatory disorders were found in individuals with ACS above 50% compared to those with ACS fewer than 50% and without carotid atherosclerosis (p < 0.05).

Our longitudinal population-based neurosonographic study revealed that the incidence of hemodynamically insignificant and hemodynamically significant ACS increased with the age. For the two years period of follow up the incidence of hemodynamically significant stenoses increased from 6.4% to 7.4% and the incidence of hemodynamically insignificant stenoses from 54.6% to 57.9%. The larger number of individuals with ACS at

the second observation was possibly related to the increase in the relative part of individuals above 60 years of age in our population (49.2% at the first investigation and 58.6% at the second one). In hemodynamically significant ACS a regression in their degree was found in 12.5% which was also observed in studies using cerebral angiography (Chaturvedi S et al. 1994). In 15.6% of the stenoses above 50%, a progression in the degree of the stenosis had occurred. Similar results were also obtained in other studies using ultrasound techniques but they were not population-based (Mansour MA et al. 1999; Muluk SC et al. 1999).

In 9.4% of the hemodynamically significant ACS, a homolateral ischemic cerebral circulatory disorder had occurred. The incidence of ischemic strokes for the two years period of study for these stenoses was 3.13%. It differed from the reported from other studies higher incidence of strokes (Teal PA et al. 1998; Mansour MA et al. 1999). The difference was possibly due to the patient's selection as well as to the inclusion of individuals only with high grade ACS in these studies. Our study was population-based epidemiological longitudinal and followed up individuals with stenoses above 50%.

Ischemic cerebral circulatory disorders among individuals with low grade ACS had almost the same incidence for both genders and the older age group prevailed. They are more often in the carotid system compared to the vertebro-basillar one. The risk of development of myocardial infarction is higher in men with insignificant ACS which confirmed the hypothesis that the presence of such stenoses was a sign of generalized atherosclerosis.

We found in our study that ischemic cerebral circulatory disorders were significantly higher among individuals with hemodynamically significant ACS. These results confirmed the previously published data (Norris JW et al. 1991).

Data from our longitudinal population-based neurosonographic study showed the great incidence of ACS among the investigated city residents of age 50-79 and confirmed the need of using ultrasound techniques in the general strategy for prophylaxis of TIA'S and ischemic stroke.

5.1.5. *Diabetes mellitus*

The incidence of diabetes mellitus in our country has been constantly increasing from 0.2% at the beginning of the previous century to 2.07% in the last years (Merdganov Ch 1995). Austrian-Bulgarian epidemiological study of cerebrovascular RFs found that distribution of diabetes mellitus was the same for the Austrian and Bulgarian population and accounted to 6.5% (Lechner H, Hadgjiev D 1998e).

Diabetes mellitus among men (8.7%) and among women (9.2%) in the age subgroup between 60 and 79 years was more frequent compared to the subgroup between 50 and 59 years, respectively 1.0% and 3.2% ($p < 0.05$).

The trend to increase in the incidence of diabetes mellitus with the increase of the age was observed at the second study, too. The rates of this well documented RF for stroke were higher among the investigated individuals from both genders in the age interval of 60-79 years where it was respectively 9.9% for men and 10.2% for women at the second study, too. This incidence was statistically significantly higher than the reported among the younger age group ($p < 0.05$).

Distribution of diabetes mellitus increased for both genders with the increase of the age. Its rates at the second study were higher compared to the first one (**Fig. 7**).

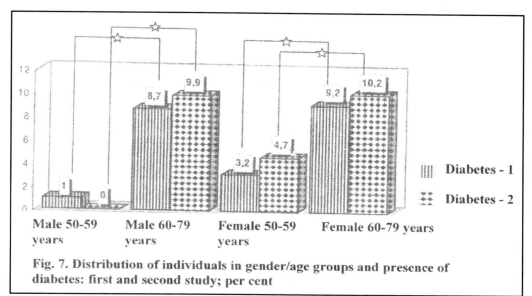

Figure 7

Fig. 7. Distribution of individuals in gender/age groups and presence of diabetes: first and second study; per cent

The incidence of diabetes mellitus among the investigated by our staff individuals was similar to that of the two populations from the Austrian-Bulgarian study (Lechner H, Hadgjiev D 1998f).

The incidence of diabetes mellitus showed differences in the different ethnic groups. Population-based cohort study held in Finland among 10, 622 diabetic patients found big differences in the development of ischemic strokes and cardiac infarctions in two separate ethnic groups (Njolstad I et al. 1998) and prospective cohort study held in Scotland including 366, 849 individuals found that the incidence of diabetes mellitus was 2.1% (Donnan PT et al. 2000).

Cases of type II diabetes mellitus prevailed in our epidemiological study which more often caused ischemic stroke occurrence. These data were obtained from the most of the studies although there were observations confirming the role of type I diabetes mellitus which also led to development of strokes (Fulesdi B et al. 1997).

Atherothrombotic strokes are more often in diabetes mellitus compared to subarachnoid and cerebral hemorrhages (Mankovsky BN et al. 1996; Hadgjiev D 1987). Our study did not register subarachnoid and cerebral hemorrhages but only TIA'S and cerebral infarctions. In both cases of cerebral infarction was found a combination of two well documented RFs for CVD - diabetes mellitus and hemodynamically significant ACS.

In most of the cases hyperglycemia increased the risk for development of ischemic stroke (Sharma AK et al. 1996; Steingrub JS, Mundt DJ 1996; Nagi M et al. 1999). On the other hand, the systemic control over blood sugar lowered the risk for a new stroke (Alter M et al. 1997; UK Prospective Diabetes Study Group 1998). This imposed the need to carry out systemic screening investigations of large groups of risk populations with respect to prevention of the diabetic complications including cerebrovascular diseases.

Data from our longitudinal population-based epidemiological study indicated high incidence of diabetes mellitus especially with the increase of the age of healthy individuals. Although in most of the cases diabetes mellitus was combined with other well and less well documented RFs for CVD, it was necessary to conduct systemic epidemiological studies for detection of hyperglycemia and latent forms of diabetes with respect to the their in time treatment by means of a diet and

increase in the motion activity of the risk groups. On its turn, this would give the opportunity to prevent vascular complications which would have occurred after a certain period of time.

5.2. Less well documented risk factors for CVD

5.2.1. Hyperlipidemia

Bulgarian authors have studied in details the role of hypercholesterolemia and hyperlipoproteinemia as risk factors for cardiovascular diseases. Studies held in our country indicated that hypercholesterolemia among the population above 40 years of age was 16%. The values of this parameter were highest in men under 50 years of age and in women above this age. Besides, it was found that concentrations of serum cholesterol statistically significantly increased with the increase of body weight, arterial hypertension, alcohol abuse and smoking and also with increased consumption of animal fat (Merdganov Ch 1995). Austrian-Bulgarian comparative population-based study showed that hypercholesterolemia was more frequent among the investigated Bulgarian population – 41.7% than among Austrian – 31.7%. Elevation of triglycerides was found with approximately same frequency in both groups of investigated individuals – 16.2% and respectively, 17.2% (Lechner H, Hadgjiev D 1998g).

The increase of total cholesterol in the age group 50-59 years was more frequent for women – 21.0% compared to men – 10.5% ($p < 0.01$). Even more expressed were the differences between the two genders of the age 60-79 for which the hypercholesterolemia was respectively 17% for the women and 4.8% for the men ($p < 0.001$).

Pathologic abnormalities of HDL were more frequent among men of the age subgroup 60-79 -24.0% compared
to the women of the same age – 6.3% ($p < 0.001$). The values of this parameter also were higher among men of the age subgroup 50-59 -17.9% compared to the women – 12.7% but the differences between them were statistically insignificant.

Most frequently the values of LDL were elevated in men and women from the age subgroup of 60-79 (77.8%). In this case, the abnormal values did not statistically significantly differ in the different age subgroups.

At the second study, abnormally increased triglycerides were found most frequently in men of the age 50-59 – 34.8% and most rarely in women of the age subgroup 60-79 – 17.4%. The differences in the values of this parameter did not significantly vary between each other both by gender and by age.

Distribution of individuals with increased cholesterol by gender and age found in the first and second investigation is represented in **Figure 8**.

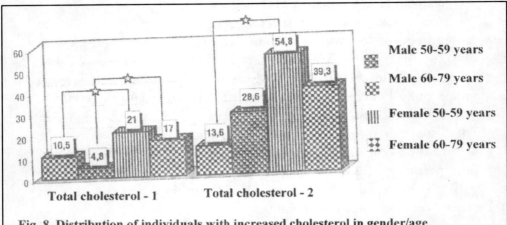

Fig. 8. Distribution of individuals with increased cholesterol in gender/age groups: first and second study; per cent

It was seen from the figure that the number of individuals with abnormal cholesterol in the second study increased but without the differences between them to be statistically significant. The incidence of hypercholesterolemia in the investigated healthy individuals was lower than the reported in the two populations from Austrian-Bulgarian study (Lechner H, Hadgjiev D 1998h). Another study held in our country found an incidence of hypercholesterolemia respectively 17% for men and 14% for women of the age group above 40 (Merdganov Ch 1995). The role of cholesterol as a RF for CVD was pointed out in a number of studies (Jacobs DR 1994; Stoy NS 1997; Dykers AG et al. 1997) and in other ones was taken into account its combined effect together with other risk factors for cardiovascular and cerebrovascular diseases like hypertension, smoking, impaired rheologic properties of the blood, increased blood sugar, etc. (Florkowski CM et al. 1998; Honczarenko K et al. 1999; Leppala JM et al. 1999; Beckett N et al. 2000; Mannami T et al. 2000).

Compared to ischemic cerebral circulatory disorders, the increase of total cholesterol showed a feedback to the cerebral hemorrhages incidents – RR 2.7 (95% Cl 1.4 to 5.0) (Giroud M et al. 1995; Irribaren C et al. 1996; Ozawa H et al. 1996).

High values of cholesterol and lipoproteins account to progression of the carotid atherosclerosis (Chen WH et al. 1996; Postorino G et al. 1996; Wilson PW et al. 1997; Pan WH et al. 1997; Goff DC et al. 2000).

On the contrary to the pointed data, a number of epidemiological studies showed that there was no relation between the level of plasma cholesterol and strokes or that this relation was unconvincing (Jacobs DR 1994; Stoy NS 1997).

Pathologic abnormalities of HDL were more frequent in our population especially among men of the age 60-79 compared to the populations from Austrian-Bulgarian study (**Figure 9**).

Figure 9

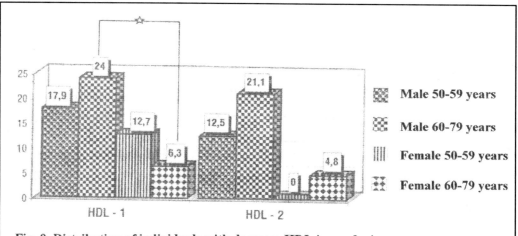

Fig. 9. **Distribution of individuals with decrease HDL in gender/age groups:** first and second study; per cent

At our second investigation a statistically significant decrease of HDL was registered during the second observation compared to the first one. This change was present for both age groups ($p < 0.001$). The protective action of HDL against the occurrence of strokes was pointed out by a number of authors (Sich D et al. 1998; Wannamethee SG et al. 2000).

The incidence of the increased LDL in our study was lower than that of Austrian and Bulgarian populations (**Figure 10**).

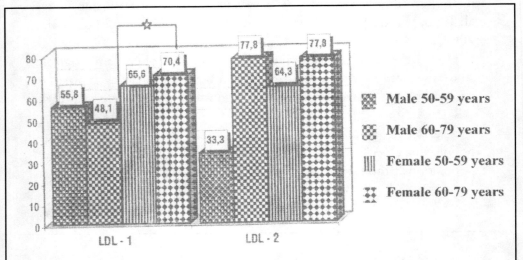

Fig. 10. Distribution of individuals with increased LDL in gender/age groups: first and second study; per cent

At the second observation, a statistically significant increase in the incidences of this parameter was registered compared to the first one.

Except that it was a risk factor fro stroke, the increased LDL provides the option fro progression of carotid atherosclerosis (Hodis HN et al. 1997; Landray MG et al. 1998).

Hypertriglyceridemia was lower at our study than the reported from both populations of Austrian-Bulgarian study (**Figure 11**).

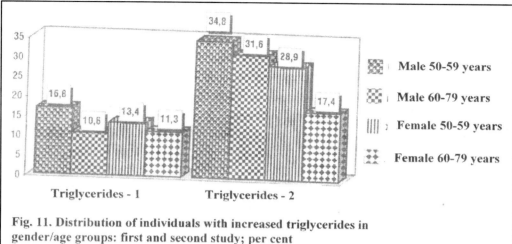

Fig. 11. Distribution of individuals with increased triglycerides in gender/age groups: first and second study; per cent

Its incidence increased insignificantly during the second observation compared to the background study. Parallel clinical Doppler and biochemical investigations revealed that the increased triglycerides were a frequent RF for strokes and carotid atherosclerosis (Kowal P 1995; Gronholdt MT et al. 1998; Gerivaise N et al. 2000).

There is a lot of evidence that high values of total plasma cholesterol, LDL and serum triglycerides are statistically significantly more frequent in patients with atherothrombic strokes and in TIA'S compared to the control group of healthy individuals (Zuber M, Mas JL 1994; Kowal P 1995; Aull S et al. 1996; Hachinski V et al. 1996; Leonardt G, Diener HC 1996; Catalano M et al. 1998; Papadakis JA et al. 1998; Albucher Jf et al. 2000; Mfrtando RM 2000).

Via studies conducted we assessed the dependence between pathologic abnormalities of lipid parameters and the other analyzed RFs for CVD. It was found that there was dependence between hypercholesterolemia and blood sugar level. Also significant was the dependence between hypertriglyceridemia and overweight. The relation between the investigated lipid parameters and other RFs – systolic and diastolic pressure, smoking, fibrinogen and hematocrit- was statistically insignificant.

Our study showed that hypercholesterolemia and hypertriglyceridemia were statistically significantly associated with blood sugar level and respectively with overweight. These dependences also were the argumentation of some therapeutic effects in dyslipidemia – normalization of blood sugar and body weight. The lack of dependences towards the rest of analyzed by our staff RFs for CVD revealed that dyslipidemia could be independent treatable risk factor.

All these results showed the need of conduction of new longitudinal epidemiological studies for define more accurately the role of dyslipidemia in the pathogenesis of cerebrovascular diseases. This was necessary for the fact that successful therapeutic effect on arterial hypertension in the last years in Western European countries and the USA did not lead to significant decrease of morbidity and mortality of strokes. This revealed that the role of less well documented cerebreovascular RFs, dyslipidemia in this case, was possibly more significant. Therefore, the prophylaxis of CVD should be focused not only against arterial hypertension but also against hyperlipidemia.

5.2.2. Use of oral contraceptives

A number of clinical trials showed that the use of oral contraceptives increased the risk of ischemic stroke development but there were only single reports dedicated to this issue in our country (Hadgjiev D et al. 1985).

At the first observation only 7 (1.4%) of the investigated women had used oral contraceptives in different periods of their lives. Due to the older age of the participants in the study, it was possible that the percentage of oral contraceptives users was insignificant.

At the second study no new data about the use of oral contraceptives was obtained from the investigated by our staff populations of women aged 50-59 and 60-69.

Result analysis from the study of oral contraceptives showed that women who had used these medicinal products did not suffer strokes. However, the small number of observations did not allow us to make general conclusions.

It is known that oral contraceptives carry out a risk for ischemic stroke development mainly at present thrombosis of cerebral arteries, veins and dural sinuses which was pointed out in a number of standard and case-control studies (Heinemann LA et al. 1997; Lidegaard O, Kreiner S 1998; Heinemann LA 2000; Godsland IF et al. 2000).

In most of the cases the impact of oral contraceptives was combined with other risk factors like smoking, arterial hypertension, dyslipidemia, overweight and age above 35 (Levin SR et al. 1991; Hannaford PC et al. 1994; Heinemann LA et al. 1998; Lidegaard O 1999; Farley TM et al. 1999).

In such combination of RFs the options ratios for stroke occurrence increased significantly – OR 3.6 (95% Cl, 2.4 to 5.4).

Prospective cohort case-control studies found that the relative risk for development of ischemic strokes, subarachnoid and cerebral hemorrhages for women using oral contraceptives increased from 0.6 to 2.5 (Thorogood M et al. 1992; WHO Coll. Study 1999; Mhurchu CN et al. 2001).

However, other epidemiological studies revealed that the use of oral contraceptives, containing low doses of estrogen, did not enhance the risk for stroke (WHO Coll. Study 1996; Jonston SC et al. 1998; Zeitoun K, Carr BR 1999; Bousser MG, Kittner SJ 2000).

The controversial results obtained from clinical-epidemiological studies dedicated to the impact of using oral contraceptives and their relation to ischemic strokes necessitate detailed investigations in order to exclude the influence of other RFs for CVD. Therefore, at the presence of other risk factors for stroke it was recommended not to use these medicinal products especially by women of age above 40.

5.2.3. Alcohol abuse

Epidemiology of alcoholism in Bulgaria was studied in details by Uzunov G et al. (1961), Stankushev T (1977, 1990) (by Merdganov Ch 1995).

It was found that arterial hypertension, smoking and alcohol abuse were significantly more often among men compared to women (Hadgjiev D 1998).

At the first observation alcohol abuse was found most frequently among men of age 50-59 (13.5%) followed by the reported one of the older men (9.6%). Their rates appeared statistically significantly higher compared to those of the women from both age subgroups in which alcohol abuse was not found ($p < 0.0001$).

At the second study, no essential differences in the rates of alcohol abuse among men were registered but a slight increase in the incidence of this parameter among men of age 60-79 (11.9%) was detected. In that case, the rates of alcohol abuse among men were significantly higher compared to those of the women from both age subgroups (p < 0.0001).

The dynamics of the rates of alcohol abuse for both studies is represented in **Figure 12**.

Figure 12

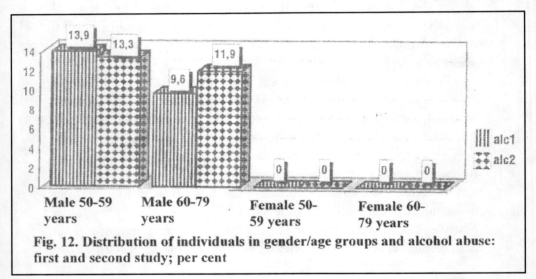

Fig. 12. Distribution of individuals in gender/age groups and alcohol abuse: first and second study; per cent

The result analysis showed that no essential changes in the rates of alcohol abuse for both studies had occurred.

The incidence of alcohol abuse reported for our population was close to the one detected by other Bulgarian authors (Merdganov Ch 1995) with the difference those women from the investigated by our staff age subgroups of 50-59 and 60-79 did not abuse with alcohol.

Framingham study revealed that the relation between alcohol consumption and strokes was possibly present only in men and alcohol abuse was frequently in combination with arterial hypertension and smoking. However, a number of trials including some case-control studies indicated that alcohol abuse was a risk factor for stroke in women, too (Bradley KA et al. 1998; Caycoya M et al. 1999).

The changes in the values of arterial pressure, HDL and platelet aggregation appeared to be dependant on alcohol consumption in coronary heart diseases but such relation was not found for cerebrovascular diseases (Numminen H et al. 2000; De Lorimier AA 2000). The risk for strokes was investigated in population of 26, 556 men who were smokers of age 50-69 and without past history of preceding stroke incidents. Following subgroups were formed: individuals who did not drink alcohol, individuals who drank small amounts (< 24 g daily), moderate amounts (from 25 g to 60 g daily) and large amounts (60 g daily) of alcohol. The relative risk for stroke was respectively 0.9:1.2:1.5. Systolic arterial pressure decreased the effect of alcohol consumption in all types of stroke while HDL enhanced this effect in subarachnoid haemorrhages and reduced it in intracerebral haemorrhages (Leppala MJ et al. 1996). The relative risk for development of subarachnoid haemorrhages in men and women using large amounts of alcohol accounted to 4.3 (95% Cl, 1.1 to 16.8) and if the alcohol abuse was combined with smoking and arterial hypertension this risk increased to 6.0 (95% Cl, 1.8 to 20.0) (Sankai H et al. 2000).

Consumption of large amounts of alcohol showed a relation to the progression of atherosclerotic process and increase of the arterial pressure values and according to some authors, consumption of small amounts of alcohol might have a protective effect (Kiechl S et al. 1998; Campbell NR et al. 1999).

The relative risk for fatal outcome for individuals who consumed large amounts of alcohol accounted to 1.74 while for those who did not consume it was 1.34 (Harf CL et al. 1999). The favourable effect on stroke mortality was not registered also in individuals using moderate amounts of alcohol (Meister KA et al. 2000).

Prevailing part of epidemiological studies provides the argumentation to assume that chronic alcohol abuse is a risk factor for strokes. However, data concerning cerebral infarctions is still controversial especially consuming small and moderate amounts of alcohol.

5.2.4. Obesity

Earlier epidemiological observations in our country indicated that obesity was one of the most widely spread RF for cardiac and cerebrovascular diseases. It was found that the obesity incidence had increased several times in a number of country regions in the last decades (Merdganov Ch 1995). Austrian-Bulgarian comparative population-based study revealed that this RF for CVD among the age groups of 49-74 was observed with approximately the same frequency in Austrian and Bulgarian populations, respectively 38.8% and 36.3% (Lechner H, Hadgjiev D 1996). Population-based epidemiological study of cerebrovascular risk factors held in our country found that BMI above 27.3 kg/m^2 was observed in 41.4% of all the investigated individuals. Its values were usually increased among women of age 60-79 (50.7%) and 50-59 (43.9%) (Hadgjiev D et al. 1999).

The obesity incidence was highest among women of the age interval 60-79 (50.7%). It differed statistically significantly from the reported one for the male population of the same age ($p < 0.001$). Higher BMI was observed also in younger women compared to that of men of the same age interval but without the differences in their incidences to be statistically significant.

At the second observation obesity was again most frequent among women of age 60-79 (54.2%). Its incidence was statistically higher than that reported in men of the same age – 34.2% ($p < 0.001$). Obesity was

insignificantly more common women of age 50-59 compared to men of the same age group.

Dynamic follow up of the obesity incidence showed increase with the increase of the age. Besides, the incidences of this RF were increased among women compared to men in both age groups (**Figure 13**).

Figure 13

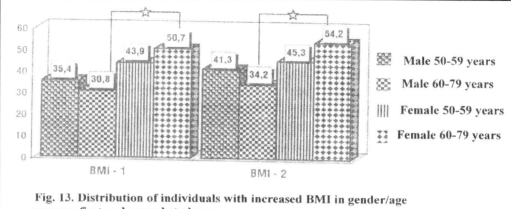

Fig. 13. Distribution of individuals with increased BMI in gender/age groups: first and second study; per cent

The rates of overweight found in our population were similar to that of Austrian and Bulgarian populations from Austrian-Bulgarian study (Lechner H, Hadgjiev D 1998k).

Abdominal obesity was a significant RF for development of myocardial and cerebral infarction and increased significantly the possibility of lethal outcome from these diseases (Megnien JL et al. 1999). Other similar to our investigation studies also found that a higher incidence of obesity in women compared to men. In such study was found that obesity was a RF for the occurrence of new atherothrombotic cerebral infarction among old women while in men from the same age its impact was

insignificant (Aronow WS et al. 1996). Beside, high BMI increased the risk for occurrence of cerebral haemorrhage (Xu WL et al. 1994).

Some data indicated that increased BMI (above 27 kg/m^2) reduced the risk for fatal respiratory disease but increased the risk for cardiovascular and cerebrovascular diseases among women who had never smoked (Singh PN, Lindsted KD 1998).

Obesity combined with arterial hypertension and hyperlipidemia was found in individuals exposed to continuous stress (Kadojiyc D et al. 1998).

Overweight usually combined with other RFs for CVD. Study held among the African population found that the incidence of obesity

(44.2%) followed immediately after poorly controlled hypertension (83.9%), then hyperlipidemia (20.6%), smoking (12.4%), hypercholesterolemia (8.1%) and diabetes mellitus (7.3%) (Zabsorne P et al. 1997).

Large epidemiological study called The Atherosclerosis Risk in Communities Study (ARIC) involving 13, 282 men and women of age 45-64 revealed that high body weight was a RF for the development and intensification of atheromatous changes in carotid arteries (Stevens J et al. 1998).

Recently by means of population-based case-control epidemiological study and multivariate analysis method was found that hypertension, left ventricular hypertrophy diagnosed by ECG investigation, ischemic heart disease, mitral valve diseases, regular smoking and high BMI were significant and independent RFs for stroke (Feigin VL et al. 1998).

Despite the controversial opinions about the role of obesity as an independent RF for ischemic stroke, its impact could be considered proven. Therefore, the normalization of overweight should be included in the complex prophylactic programs for limitation of cerebrovascular and cardiovascular diseases.

5.2.5. Increased hematocrit

Haemorrheological studies were held among individuals with latent, transient and chronic cerebral circulatory insufficiency which showed higher values of hematocrit and fibrinogen compared to the control group of healthy individuals (Velcheva I, Boeva D 1993). The role of impaired rheological blood properties in CVD was marked by other Bulgarian authors, too (Manchev I 2001) but so far there were no longitudinal epidemiological studies about their impact held in our countries.

At the first study conducted among 500 healthy individuals of age 50-79 increased values of hematocrit were found in 5 (1%) of them. Increased hematocrit were detected among the age group 50-59 for both gender.

At the conducted in two years second observation of the same population and by means of the same methods increased hematocrit was found in only one man (1.8%) of the age interval 60-79.

A number of trials were dedicated to the relation of hematocrit and fibrinogen to cardiovascular and cerebrovascular diseases. Increasing of blood and plasma viscosity which was determined by the increase of hematocrit and fibrinogen values usually led to development of ischemic heart disease and stroke (Resch

KL, Erust E 1990; Grobbee DE et al. 1996; Love GD et al. 1997; Tsuda Y et al. 1997; Woodward M et al. 1999).

The increase of hematocrit especially when it was combined with arterial hypertension carried out a high

risk for stroke development (RR 2.9 95% Cl 2.2 to 3.7) (Banerjee R et al. 2000).

Smoking, increased BMI, reduced physical activity, alcohol abuse and high serum lipid levels are factors strongly associated with hematocrit levels without being related to each other.

Their combination increased significantly the risk for ischemic stroke (Vincent M et al. 1996; Jorgensen HS et al. 1997). Hematocrit levels were statistically significantly higher among smokers of both genders compared to non-smokers. Besides, men smokers consumed large amounts of meat and tea. BMI was higher in individuals smoking more than 25 cigarettes daily (Beser E et al. 1995).

In most of the cases hematocrit levels were associated with lots of other pathologic processes – arterial hypertension, cardiovascular diseases and diabetes mellitus as well as with some other vascular risk factors like smoking, alcohol abuse, hypodynamic lifestyle, etc. The small number of individuals with increased hematocrit in our study did not allow making conclusions about its impact on the formation of various types of cerebral circulatory disorders. This defined the necessity of conducting new larger studies dedicated to this risk factor.

5.2.6. Reduced physical activity

Motion immobilization of the Bulgarian population was investigated in details by our authors. Among all the studies dedicated to this issue, three large studies were outstanding and were held according to the international criteria for assessment – Yanev B et al. 1961, 1972; Slunchev P et al. 1982 (Merdganov Ch 1995). Other carried out epidemiological studies in our country found that after 15 years of age motion activity of the population continuously worsened and the parameters of motion activity in women were more unfavorable (Merdganov Ch 1995). Austrian-Bulgarian comparative population-based epidemiological study of CRF found that reduced physical activity among individuals between 49 and 74 years of age was more frequent among the Austrian compared to Bulgarian population, respectively 38% and 17.8% (Lechner H, Hadgjiev D 1996k).

At the first study reduced physical activity was most popular among women of age 60-79 (19.7%), followed by the reported in men of age 50-59 (15.6%) and most rarely motion inactivity was detected in the subgroup of younger women (8.2%).

The incidence of this risk factor among older women appeared to be statistically significantly higher compared to the younger one ($p < 0.05$).

At the control study reduced physical activity was most popular among women of age 60-79 (19.8%) and in younger men (15.7%). The incidence of this risk was again significantly higher among women of age 60-79 compared to those of the age subgroup 50-59 (7.6%) ($p < 0.05$).

Figure 14 represents the distribution of individuals with reduced physical activity by gender and age at the first and second study. A significant increase of motion inactivity was found for the period of two years.

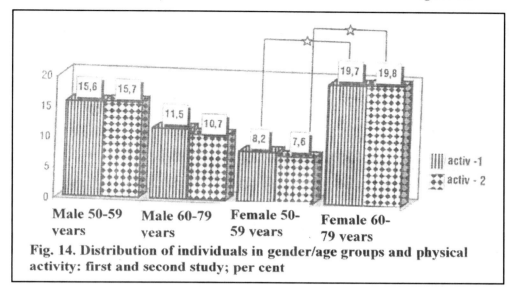

Fig. 14. Distribution of individuals in gender/age groups and physical activity: first and second study; per cent

Reduced physical activity among the investigated by our staff healthy individuals was closer to the reported for the Bulgarian city population and was lower than the reported one for the Austrian population (Hadgjiev D, Lechner H 1996k).

The role of reduced physical activity for the development of stroke was a subject of a number of other studies, too (Ellekjaer E et al. 1992; Wannamethee G et al. 1992). Data from Framingham cohort showed the relation between the sedentary lifestyle and stroke morbidity but the difference compared to the control group was statistically insignificant (Dyken ML et al. 1984).

Prospective 15.5-year epidemiological study assessed the risk factors for stroke in the Japanese population. Multivariate analysis realized by proportional random Cox-model determined the following risk factors as statistically significant for all types of stroke:

⇨ For men: age, blood pressure, atrial fibrillation, albuminuria, vascular changes of the ocular fundus, smoking and extreme physical activity.

⇨ For women: age, atrial fibrillation and mild physical activity.

But physical activity for both genders was not a RF for cerebral infarction (Nakayama T et al. 1997).

On the other hand, moderate physical activity exerted protective effect on lowering blood pressure, obesity and diabetes mellitus and therefore, reduced the risk for stroke (Claeroux J et al. 1999; Gariballa SE 2000).

Data from carried out population-based epidemiological studies no matter what were the differences in the assessment criteria revealed that moderate physical activity should be included in the complex prophylaxis of ischemic strokes.

5.2.7. Migraine

Single reports have been published in our country treating the role of migraine for manifestation of cerebral infarctions (Hadgjiev D et al. 1996) but epidemiological studies dedicated to this problem are missing.

At performing the first stage of our study migraine was found in 9 individuals. Most frequently this risk factor was detected in women of age 50-59 (4.7%). This frequency happened to be statistically significantly higher compared to the reported for men of the same age ($p < 0.05$). Migraine was not found in men of age 60-79 and in the rest of the subgroups there was one patient in each of them.

At the second observation held in two years, migraine was again most popular among younger women but without the differences in the incidences of the different age-gender subgroups to be statistically significant.

Our longitudinal epidemiological study of CRF found 9 clinical cases of migraine which accounted to 2% of the total of 500 investigated healthy individuals of age 50-79. Due to the small number of cases, it could not be declared for certain that in those cases migraine was the reason for manifestation of cerebral infarctions in our population.

The importance of migraine as a risk factor for cerebral infarctions is still under discussion. A number of reports are known which demonstrate its role in the ischemic stroke occurrence (Welch KM 1994; Tzourio C, Bousser MG 1997; Merikangas KR et al. 1997).

Population-based epidemiological studies found that stroke morbidity of migraine patients was very low: for women it accounted to 1.02 of 100, 000 populations and for men was 0.57 of 100, 000 populations (Sochurkova D et al. 1999). Besides, migraine in young women usually combined with other RFs for CVD like smoking, oral contraceptives, hypertension, and presence of anticardiolipin antibodies (Leira R, Tietjen GE 2000). Cerebral infarctions were more frequent in the presence of reduced physical activity and tension headache in men (Rasmussen BK 1993).

Of interest was the fact that cerebral infarction was significantly more frequent in patients with migraine with aura compared to those when migrainous attacks were not preceded by aura (Narbone MC et al. 1996; Tzourio C, Bousser MG 2000; Tzourio C et al. 2000).

Case-control study held among 72 women with migraine and cerebral infarction and control group of 172 women of the same age found statistically significant relationship between the presences of migraine and ischemic strokes. In women with migraine with preceding aura the options ratio were higher (OR 6.2 95% Cl 2.1 to 18.0) compared to migraine without aura (OR 3.0 95% Cl 1.5 to 5.8) (Tzourio C et al. 1995). Other case-control study held among 291 women of age

20 to 44 with ischemic, haemorrhagic and non-classified stroke and control group of 736 women of the same age found that strokes were more frequent at the presences of migraine with aura (OR 3.81 95% Cl 1.26 to 11.5) compared to cases without aura (OR 2.97 95% Cl 0.66 to 13.5) (Chang CL et al. 1999).

Despite the published results from the studies of numerous authors about the role of migraine as an etiological factor for stroke, determination of migraine as a basic RF should be done after excluding the influence of the other CRF as leading ones. In reference to that new larger epidemiological studies in women of younger age are needed.

5.3. Combination of risk factors for CVD

A lot of Bulgarian authors have studied combinations between the different risk factors and first of all, in the development of ischemic heart disease but only few investigations have been dedicated to the combination of risk factors for CVD – Ganev G et al. (1974, 1975), Gachev G (1987) (by Merdganov Ch 1995). Recently, a population-based epidemiological study about the multiple cerebrovascular risk factors was held among 500 healthy individuals of age 50-69 (Hadgjiev et al. 1999).

At our study the analyzed treatable RFs were defined as multiple in combination of four or more of them. The incidence and structure of well and less well documented multiple RFs and their combinations marked as mixed multiple RFs were separately examined. The incidence of multiple RFs was analyzed also with respect to the age and gender of the investigated individuals.

Only well documented RFs were found in 64 of the investigated individuals. One or two RFs were detected in 73.5% of them. In 8 (12.5%) individuals from this group the well documented RFs were multiple.

Single less well documented RFs were registered in 111 of the investigated individuals. Individuals with one or two RFs from this group constitute 84.7%. Multiple less well documented RFs were found in 6 (5.4%) of the observed volunteers.

Single well and less well documented RFs were found in 2.8% of the investigated individuals and multiple mixed RFs in 33.6% of them. Multiple CRFs from the three groups were registered in 180 (36%) of the investigated individuals.

There were no statistically significant differences between the incidences of multiple RFs among the investigated men and women from the two age groups. The differences in the incidences of multiple RFs between the two age groups among the investigated men and women and totally for both genders were also statistically insignificant.

The analysis of the five combinations of single multiple well documented RFs determined by our study showed that all included systolic and diastolic hypertension, three – cardiovascular diseases and smoking and two – diabetes mellitus and hemodynamically significant ACS.

Single multiple well documented RFs were represented in two combinations. They included dyslipidemias and overweight and in one of the combinations HDL reduction was missing.

The incidence of the different RFs in the group of individuals with mixed CRF is showed in **Figure 15**.

Figure 15

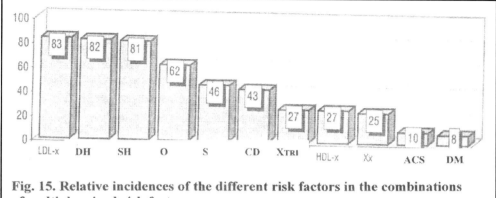

Fig. 15. Relative incidences of the different risk factors in the combinations of multiple mixed risk factors

Legend:

LDL-x – increase of LDL; DX - diastolic hypertension;
CX - systolic hypertension; HT – overweight; T – smoking;
C3 – cardiovascular diseases; Xtri – hypertriglyceridemia;
HDL-x – decrease of HDL; Xx – hypercholesterolemia;
AKC - hemodynamically significant carotid stenoses;
3D – diabetes mellitus.

Increase of LDL, diastolic and systolic hypertension, and overweight were found most frequent. Smoking and cardiovascular diseases were registered in 46% and respectively in 43% of the investigated in this group. The incidences of decreased HDL and hypertriglyceridemia were identical – 27%. Hypercholesterolemia was found in 25% of the investigated individuals. The smallest was the relative part of hemodynamically significant ACS (10%) and diabetes mellitus (8%).

The combinations of multiple mixed CRF were 90. The relative incidences of the different RFs participating in them are represented in **Figure 16**.

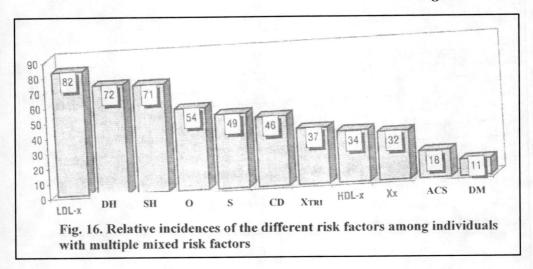

Fig. 16. Relative incidences of the different risk factors among individuals with multiple mixed risk factors

Legend:

LDL-x – increase of LDL; DH - diastolic hypertension;
CX - systolic hypertension; HTT – overweight; T – smoking;
C3 – cardiovascular diseases; Xtri – hypertriglyceridemia;
HDL-x – decrease of HDL; Xx – hypercholesterolemia;
AKC - hemodynamically significant carotid stenoses;
ЗД – diabetes mellitus.

Increased LDL (82%), diastolic (72%) and systolic hypertension (71%), and overweight (54%) had the highest relative incidences. These RFs constituted more than a half of the combinations of multiple mixed RF. Smoking and cardiovascular diseases were added in 49% and respectively 46% of the observed combinations of RF. Hypertriglyceridemia and hypercholesterolemia consisted 37% and respectively 36% of the identified combinations and decreased HDL was in 34% of them.

The smallest was the relative part of hemodynamically significant ACS (18%) and diabetes mellitus (11%).

With the current population-based epidemiological study of the treatable CRF was found that combinations of four and more than four RFs defined as multiple were detected in 36% of the investigated

500 individuals of age 50 to 79. Single multiple well or less well documented RFs were found in 1.6% and respectively in 1.2% of the investigated population.

The greatest was the incidence of multiple mixed RFs in which well and less well documented ones combined. They were registered in 33.6% of the individuals included in the study.

No statistically significant differences were found between the incidences of the multiple RFs among the investigated men and women from the two age groups.

In the separate combinations of multiple CRFs there was a prevalence of systolic and diastolic hypertension, dyslipidemias, overweight, smoking and cardiovascular diseases. Less frequent were hemodynamically significant ACS and diabetes mellitus. The great incidence of multiple CRFs suggested that their carriers should be the target of complex primary prophylaxis directed against all treatable RFs and especially against those of them associated with the lifestyle.

Austrian-Bulgarian epidemiological study found that the CRF distribution in the Bulgarian population was greater than in the Austrian one. Besides, the combinations of three and more RFs were more frequent in the Bulgarian population (Lechner K, Hadgjiev D 1998; Lechner H et al. 1999).

In some earlier studies the combination of arterial hypertension, smoking and lower parameter of the individual height and weight ratio was associated with

higher risk for fatal strokes (Paffenbarger RS, Williams JL 1967). The risk for strokes increased 12.5 times when arterial hypertension was combined with ischemic heart disease and diabetes mellitus and there was a family predisposition for arterial hypertension (Paffenbarger RS, Wing AL 1971).

Framingham longitudinal epidemiological study showed that the combination of arterial hypertension, hypercholesterolemia, and diabetes mellitus, smoking and left ventricular hypertrophy known as Framingham profile enhanced the possibility of stroke. Framingham profile allowed identification of 10% of the population without manifested symptoms of CVD among which for a period of eight years had occurred half of the cerebral infarctions for the whole population (Kannel Wb 1976).

The combination of arterial hypertension with smoking, atrial fibrillation, diabetes mellitus, obesity increased the relative risk for stroke (95% Cl, 1.7 to 6.3) (Mast H et al. 1997; Du H et al. 2000). These data revealed that arterial hypertension was the most important RF for strokes but its importance increased with its combining with other RFs which necessitated its systemic control. Recent data showed that the early treatment of arterial hypertension and even its borderline values might lead to sudden decrease of stroke morbidity (Fang XH et al. 1999). Despite successful treatment of arterial hypertension, the studies held in the USA indicated that stroke mortality decreased to less extent than expected. It is suggested that the reason for this was the increase of morbidity of diabetes mellitus, obesity and heart failure (Gillum RF and Sempos Ch T 1997; Yusuff HR et al. 2000).

Our study revealed that in the combination of multiple CRF except arterial hypertension a significant part had not only overweight and cardiovascular diseases but also

dyslipidemia and smoking. High incidence of dyslipidemia was found in other studies, too (Lechner H et al. 1999). These data indicated that in order to decrease stroke morbidity and mortality, side by side with arterial hypertension control it was necessary to perform systemic prophylaxis of the other RFs for CVD.

It deserved to point out that hemodynamically significant ACS participated in approximately 20% of the combinations of multiple mixed RFs which was more often than diabetes mellitus. Their role as s treatable well documented CRF was found via numerous population-based epidemiological studies. In most of the cases ACS was combined with other RFs like hypertension, diabetes mellitus, dyslipidemias, obesity and older age which increased significantly the risk for stroke and fatal outcome (Cohen SN et al. 1993; Elkers RS et al. 1996; Cronholdt ML et al. 1996; Crouse JR et al. 1996; Beks PH et al. 1997; Franklin SS et al. 1997; Yamamoft M et al. 1997; Hadgjiev A et al. 1999).

A study held in the Spanish population continuing for two years found that the risk for stroke was the highest in combining arterial hypertension and diabetes mellitus (Lado-Lado FL et al. 1996). In 18-year prospective population-based epidemiological study of the risk factors for stroke in the Japanese population the impact of several RFs like smoking, arterial hypertension, diabetes mellitus, hyperlipidemia and obesity was studied. The risk for stroke was compared when two and more RFs were combined. Stroke morbidity for older men and women was higher when combining several RFs while in young men and women there was no higher stroke morbidity in individuals with several RFs compared to those cases of combining two RFs (Lechner H et al. 1986).

Data from our longitudinal population-based epidemiological study of the multiple CRF showed that their identification and treatment gained a significant part in the primary prophylaxis of strokes. The importance of the different combinations of multiple factors as precursors of stroke and their prognostic value can be précised by means of continuous studies of large populations of healthy individuals and risk groups.

5.4. The importance of electroencephalographic deviations for the assessment of the risk for acute cerebral circulatory disorder

Electroencephalography (EEG) has not been widely used in stroke diagnosis since this diagnosis is clinical and the typical signs of this particular disease are missing on the EEG. However, acute and chronic cerebral ischemia, the oxygen and metabolite insufficiency cause different EEG changes by their characteristics and intensity.

In the acute period of stroke a reduction of the normal cerebral rhythm is usually observed and the slow wave activity prevails (Binnie CD, Prior PE 1994).

Screening studies dedicated to the individuals endangered by stroke were held in which ECG, Doppler sonographic and EEG investigations were included together with the investigated RFs for CVD. Such was the screening system CEREBRUS which was applied in 691 individuals endangered by stroke (Bodo M et al. 1995).

Parallel Doppler sonographic and EEG investigations were done for carotid stenoses in carotid endarterectomy. Significant correlations between reduced blood flow in the carotid arteries and slowed down bioelectric activity on the EEG (Arnold M et al. 1997; Balotta E et al. 1997). Similar relations were found in the EEG and SPECT investigations. There was found a relation between reduced perfusion in the ischemic region seen on SPECT investigation and the respective disorder of the slow wave activity on EEG investigation (Suruki A et al. 1996; Inui K et al. 1998; Venerri A, Caffdra P 1998).

Some components of EEG investigation were included in Stroke Probability Index which provided the opportunity to detect individuals endangered by stroke (Lechner H 1996).

Although EEG investigation was used in our country since long ago, there were no longitudinal epidemiological studies of CRF carried out by its implication (Rasheva M 1998). Pathologic EEG were more frequent in the subgroup of women of age 60-79 (14.08%). The incidence of abnormal EEG among women of age 60-79 (14.08%) turned to be statistically significantly higher compared to the registered among men of the same age ($p < 0.001$). Focal and regional changes in the EEG were found in 27 individuals (5.4%), slowed down alpha-rhythm in 17 individuals (3.4%), and diffuse slow wave changes in delta- and teta-rhythm in 6 of the investigated individuals (1.2%). There were no statistically significant correlations between EEG changes on one hand and arterial hypertension and ACS on the other. Two years after the background investigation, new EEG investigations were done of the individuals with pathologic EEG at the first examination. At the second examination usually the pathologic EEG findings were registered among women of age 50-59, followed by those of women aged 60-79. The difference in the incidences between men and women of age 60-79 were again statistically significant ($p < 0.01$).

At the control examination focal and regional changes in the EEG were found in 20 individuals (4.0%), slowed down alpha-rhythm in 8 individuals (1.6%), and diffuse slow wave changes in 7 volunteers (1.4%). Pathologic changes were not found in 5 of the investigated individuals.

Figure 17 represents the incidences of pathologic EEG changes in healthy individuals by gender and age at the first and second investigation.

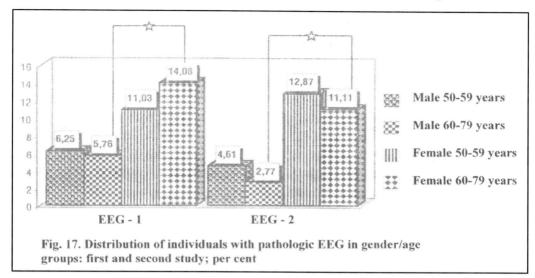

Fig. 17. Distribution of individuals with pathologic EEG in gender/age groups: first and second study; per cent

Result analysis from the two investigations did not show significance of the changes in the abnormal EEG rates for both investigations.

EEG investigations were carried out in healthy individuals of middle age with one or several CRFs. Statistically significantly more frequent focal EEG changes in patients with RF compared to the investigated individuals without such RF were found ($p < 0.05$) (Logar C et al. 1993). EEG investigations were carried out in 423 individuals with CRF. Diffuse EEG changes were detected in patients with high blood sugar and serum lipid levels, high blood pressure and cardiomyopathies (Cognazzo A et al. 1981). In the case-control study abnormal EEG was found in 14% of diabetic patients. This incidence was higher compared to the control group of healthy individuals ($p < 0.001$) (Inui K et al. 1998).

The incidence of alpha-rhythm gradually decreased in patients with cerebral atherosclerosis and vascular dementia but in return was observed increase in the percentage of slow waves, presence of transient sharp waves with temporal localization as well as frontal arrhythmia (Wilson WP et al. 1977; Zurek R et al. 1985; D'Onofrio F et al. 1996; Sato K et al. 1996).

EEG during TIA'S in the carotid system showed slow wave teta-activity at the site of the vascular incident which sometimes was mixed with sharp waves (Niedermeyer E, Da Silva FL 1987; Iyama A et al. 1992).

Epileptic seizures could appear in patients with ischemic strokes (Beaumanoir A et al. 1996) as well as temporal (Mainard SD, Hudges JR 1984; Asokan G et al. 1997) or diffuse slow wave activity (Hempel HP, Schmidt RU 1975; Yokoyama E et al. 1996; Molnar M et al. 1997; Fernandez-Bouzas A et al. 2000).

Despite its limited potentialities in the diagnostics of cerebrovascular disease, the EEG method is applicable in screening investigations of cerebrovascular RF especially when it is combined with other non-invasive techniques like Doppler sonography, SPECT and CT of the brain. Therefore, it may be included in such investigations.

SUMMARY

Our study revealed that arterial hypertension, smoking and cardiovascular diseases were the most wide spread risk factors with CVD in the investigated population. Significantly lower was the incidence of hemodynamically significant ACS and diabetes mellitus.

At the second study an increase in the incidence of arterial hypertension was found among women of both age subgroups and men aged 60-79. The increase in the incidence of AH was statistically significantly associated with the increase of the age in all the investigated groups.

Dynamic follow up of the number of individuals with systolic hypertension revealed an increase in their incidence at the second study. The increase in the number of individuals with systolic hypertension was statistically significantly associated with the increase of the age in older men and in women from both subgroups.

The incidence of diastolic hypertension also increased significantly with the increase of the age among men aged 60-79 and women from both groups.

At the first study cardiovascular diseases among men of age 60-79 were significantly more frequent compared to younger ones and compared to women of the same age interval. At the second study the incidence of cardiovascular diseases did not show a significant change compared to the background study with the exception of ischemic heart disease which increased.

Asymptomatic carotid stenoses prevailed in women from both age subgroups. Dynamic follow up of the ACS incidence by gender and age showed an insignificant increase of the number of individuals with stenoses with the increase of the age. TIA'S and cerebral infarctions developed in certain part of the patients with ACS. A statistically significantly higher incidence of these disorders was found in individuals with ACS above 50% compared to those with stenoses less than 50% and to individuals with carotid atherosclerosis.

In some of the individuals with ACS dynamically was found a progression of the stenoses and a regression of the stenoses was detected in a smaller number of individuals.

Diabetes mellitus in men and women of the age 60-79 was statistically significantly more frequent compared to the younger age group. This showed that the incidence of this risk factor increased with the increase of the age. At the second study insignificant increase of diabetes was found in all the investigated groups.

At the first study smoking showed the biggest differences concerning gender and age. It was significantly more frequent among individuals of age 50-59 for both genders. Two years after the background study this trend was preserved and the incidence of men smokers decreased while for women it almost did not change.

At the first study increased total cholesterol was statistically significantly more frequent in women from both age subgroups compared to men. At the control investigation the increased total cholesterol among women of age 50-59 was again statistically significantly more frequent compared to men from the same age interval while the incidences among women of age 60-79 were insignificantly higher compared to men of the same age.

At the first study increased LDL was significantly more frequent among women of age 60-79 compared to men of the same age while the incidences among women of age 50-59 was insignificantly higher compared to those registered in men of the same age.

Pathologic deviations of HDL at the first study were statistically significantly more frequent in men of age subgroup 60-79 compared to women of the same age while at the control observation no significant differences were found in the incidences of this parameter in the investigated population.

The values of triglycerides at the background study were insignificantly higher in men and women of age 50-59 compared to the age subgroups of 60-79. At the control observation this trend was preserved but the differences in the incidences of this RF in the different subgroups turned to be insignificant.

At the background study women of age 60-79 had more frequently overweight compared to men from the same age subgroup. This relation remained unchanged at the control observation, too.

Alcohol abuse among men from both age subgroups in both studies was statistically significantly more frequent compared to women of age 50-59 and 60-79 who did not consume alcohol.

In both studies reduced physical activity was more frequent for women of age 60-79. It turned to be significantly higher compared to the reported one for younger women.

Some less well documented RFs for CVD investigated in our study like oral contraceptives, migraine and increased hematocrit were found in a small number of the investigated individuals in both studies. Therefore, conclusions about their impact could not be drawn.

Population-based epidemiological study of the combinations of RFs for CVD held in our country found that the combinations of four and more than four RFs were registered in more than one third of the investigated healthy individuals. Single multiple well and less well documented RFs were found in a small percentage of the investigated individuals. The highest was the incidence of multiple mixed RFs in which well and less well documented RFs were combined. No statistically significant differences between the incidences of the multiple RFs among the investigated men and women from both age subgroups.

In the different combination of multiple RFs prevailed hypertension, dyslipidemias, overweight, smoking and cardiovascular diseases. At the first study pathologic EEG changes were mostly distributed among women of age 60-79. Their incidence turned to be statistically significantly higher compared to men of the same age. At the control study the incidences of pathologic EEG findings were again more frequent among older women compared to men from the same age group.

Our population-based epidemiological study found a significant distribution of the arterial hypertension whose incidence increased with the increase of the age. The incidence of this RF was similar to that of the Austrian population from the carried out the Austrian-Bulgarian study (Lechner H, Hadgjiev D 1998) as well as to that of another study in Great Britain (Kalra L et al. 1998). This incidence was higher than the reported one from the WHO ERICA Project (The WHO ERICA Project 1988) and lower than the reported one for the African population (Zabstorne P et al. 1997).

The incidences of the cardiovascular diseases and diabetes mellitus in our population was also similar to the one reported about the two populations from Austrian-Bulgarian study while smoking was significantly more widespread compared to these populations.

The incidence of hemodynamically significant ACS for all the investigated individuals was similar to the one reported by other epidemiological studies (Ricci S et al. 1991; O'Leary DH et al. 1992; Pulia A et al. 1992).

From the less well documented CRFs the incidence of hypercholesterolemia and hypertriglyceridemia was lower than the one reported for the two populations from the Austrian-Bulgarian study (Lechner H, Hadgjiev D 1998) and the documented one from the WHO ERICA Project (The WHO ERICA Project 1988). Significant geographical differences in the distribution of hypercholesterolemia were registered by the WHO MONICA Project too (Stegmayr B et al. 1997). The determined by us incidence of LDL was smaller than that in the two population from the Austrian-Bulgarian study while the pathologic deviations of HDL were more frequent in our population.

The incidence of overweight registered in our population was similar to that reported for the Austrian and Bulgarian populations from the same study.

The results from the current study confirmed wide distribution of well documented CRFs like arterial hypertension, cardiovascular diseases, and smoking. Increased LDL and overweight were also with high incidence. Compared to the other population-based epidemiological studies, some other differences in the incidences of CRFs in the investigated population by us were also marked. Registered data confirmed the presence of geographical differences in the distribution of CRFs and defined the need of their consideration in the development of stroke prophylactic programs.

REFERENCES

1. Velcheva I, Boeva D: Hemorrheological changes in cerebrovascular disease. Cerebrovascular diseases 1, 1993, 29-33
2. Vulkov J: *Ischemic heart disease - screening of the individual and population risk.* Dissertation for conferment a scientific degree "Doctor of medical sciences", Stara Zagora, 1996
3. Doichinov A: Smoking of cigarettes as a risk factor and hemostasis changes B: *Alcoholism and smoking.* Sofia, Medical Faculty, 1978, 165-169
4. Manchev I: *Clinical-epidemiological study of the latent and transient cerebral circulatory insufficiency.* Dissertation for conferment a scientific degree "Candidate of medical sciences", Sofia, 1989
5. Manchev I: Asymptomatic carotid stenoses - a risk factor for ischemic cerebral circulatory disorders. News bulletin of Stroke Prevention Foundation, 1997
6. Manchev I: Population-based epidemiological study of the cerebrovascular risk factors in Stara Zagora. Cerebrovascular diseases 2, 1999, 9-16
7. Manchev I: Transient ischemic attacks. B: Hadgjiev D, Lechner H (red.) *Ischemic strokes*, Medical Publisher "ARCO", Sofia, 2001a, 40-46
8. Manchev I: Alcohol abuse. B: Hadgjiev D, Lechner H (red.) *Ischemic strokes*, Medical Publisher "ARCO", Sofia, 2001b, 63-66
9. Manchev I: Reduced physical activity. B: Hadgjiev D, Lechner H (red.) *Ischemic strokes*, Medical Publisher "ARCO", Sofia, 2001c, 66-68
10. Manchev I: Obesity. B: Hadgjiev D, Lechner H
11. (red.) *Ischemic strokes*, Medical Publisher "ARCO", Sofia, 2001d, 68-71
12. Manchev I: Increased hematocrit and fibrinogen. B: Hadgjiev D, Lechner H (red.) *Ischemic strokes*, Medical Publisher "ARCO", Sofia, 2001e, 71-75
13. Manchev I, Mineva P: Population-based epidemiological study of hemodynamically significant carotid stenoses. Cerebrovascular diseases 2, 1998, 16-20
14. Manchev I, Mineva P: Cerebrovascular risk factors in children with asymptomatic carotid stenoses. Cerebrovascular diseases 1, 1999, 8-14

15. Mineva P, Manchev I: Distribution of asymptomatic carotid stenoses - a longitudinal population-based neurosonographic study. Cerebrovascular diseases 1, 2000, 12-16
16. Manchev I, Mineva P, Lazarova V, Nikolov N: Population-based epidemiological study of dyslipidemiae in clinically healthy adults. Cerebrovascular diseases 1, 2000, 8-11
17. Mineva P, Manchev I, Hadgjiev D: Asymptomatic carotid stenoses. B: Hadgjiev D, Lechner H (red.) *Ischemic strokes*, Medical Publisher "ARCO", Sofia, 2001, 46-51
18. Merdganov Ch: *A compromising leadership*. University Publisher "St. Climent Ohridski", Sofia, 1995
19. Merdganov Ch: Arterial hypertension in the Bulgarian risk constellation. B: *A compromising leadership*. University Publisher "St. Climent Ohridski", Sofia, 1995a, 146-173
20. Merdganov Ch: Smoking - a main reason for worsened health and preliminary death. B: *A*
21. *compromising leadership*. University Publisher "St. Climent Ohridski", Sofia, 1995b, 175-219
22. Merdganov Ch: Hypercholesterolemia in the Bulgarian risk constellation. B: *A compromising leadership*. University Publisher "St. Climent Ohridski", Sofia, 1995c, 208-219
23. Merdganov Ch: Diabetes as a socially significant disease. B: *A compromising leadership*. University Publisher "St. Climent Ohridski", Sofia, 1995d, 224-226
24. Merdganov Ch: Health risks for obesity. B: *A compromising leadership*. University Publisher "St. Climent Ohridski", Sofia, 1995e, 229-257
25. Merdganov Ch: Motion inactivity as an unhealthy factor. B: *A compromising leadership*. University Publisher "St. Climent Ohridski", Sofia, 1995f, 258-268
26. Merdganov Ch: Alcohol consumption and socially significant diseases. B: *A compromising leadership*. University Publisher "St. Climent Ohridski", Sofia, 1995g, 273-296
27. Rasheva M: Electroencephalography. B: *Cerebrovascular risk factors*, Medical Publisher "ARCO", Sofia, 1998, 118-120
28. Tomov I: *Clinical cardiology*. Sofia, Medical Faculty, 1992, 389-391
29. Torbova S: *Hypertensive disease*. Sofia, Medical Faculty, 1994
30. Feschieva D: *Contemporary epidemiology*. Publisher "Conquista", Varna, 1997
31. Hadgjiev D: Alcohol abuse. B: *Cerebrovascular risk factors*, Medical Publisher "ARCO", Sofia, 1998
32. Hadgjiev D: Risk factors for ischemic stroke. B: *Ischemic stroke*, Medical Publisher "ARCO", Sofia, 2001
33. Hadgjiev D, Vlaev S, Vassilev V: *Neuro-psychic complications of anticonception drugs*, Medical Faculty, Sofia, 1985
34. Hadgjiev D, Lechner H: *Cerebrovascular risk factors*, Medical Publisher "ARCO", Sofia, 1998

35. Hadgjiev D, Lechner H, Manchev I, Mineva P: Dyslipidemiae. B: Hadgjiev D, Lechner H (red.) *Ischemic stroke*, Medical Publisher "ARCO", Sofia, 2001a, 58-63
36. Hadgjiev D, Lechner H, Manchev I, Mineva P: Multiple risk factors. B: Hadgjiev D, Lechner H (red.) *Ischemic stroke*, Medical Publisher "ARCO", Sofia, 2001b, 82-87
37. Hadgjiev D, Manchev I: Asymptomatic carotid stenoses. B: *Cerebrovascular risk factors*, Medical Publisher "ARCO", Sofia, 1998b, 68-71
38. Hadgjiev D, Manchev I, Mineva P: Hemodynamically significant asymptomatic carotid stenoses - risk factor for cerebral ischemia. Cerebrovascular diseases 1, 1999, 5-7
39. Hadgjiev D, Manchev I, Mineva P: Multiple cerebrovascular risk factor - population-epidemiological studies. Cerebrovascular diseases 2, 1999, 16-21
40. Hadgjiev D, Manchev I, Mineva P, Lechner H: Dyslipidemia - a risk factor for ischemic stroke. Cerebrovascular diseases 1, 2000, 5-7
41. Hadgjiev D, Raichev I, Yancheva S, Petrunova V, Tityanova E: Clinical observation of migrainous cerebral infarction. Cerebrovascular diseases 4, 1996, 14-17
42. Hadgipetrova E: *The influence of smoking on cerebral hemodynamics (according to rheoencephalographic data)*. Dissertation for conferment a scientific degree "Candidate of medical sciences", Plovdiv, 1980
43. Shipkovenska E: Heart diseases. B: Hadgjiev D, Lechner H (red.) *Ischemic stroke*, Medical Publisher "ARCO", Sofia, 2001, 24-28
44. Shotekov P: Pathologic changes in the carotid system. B: *Ultrasound Doppler sonography*, Medical faculty, Sofia, 1986, 41-61
45. Shotekov P: Pathologic changes in the extracranial cerebral arteries. B: *Doppler sonography of the extracranial and peripheral arteries and veins*, Medical Publisher "Leader Press", Sofia, 1998, 91-111
46. Adler AI, Stratton IM, Neil HA, Yudkin JS, Mattews DR, Cull CA, Wright AD, Turner RC, Holman RR: Association of systolic blood pressure with macrovascular and microvascular complications of type 2 diabetes (UKPDS 3): prospective observational study. BMJ 12, 2000, 412-419
47. Albers GW: Atrial fibrillation and stroke. Three new studies, three remaining questions. Arch Intern Med 154, 1994, 1443-1448
48. Albers GW, Bittar N, Young L, Httemer CR, Gandhi AJ, Kemp SM, Hall EA, Morton OJ, Yim J, Vlasses PH: Clinical characteristics and management of acute stroke in patients with atrial fibrillation admitted to US university hospitals. Neurology 48, 1997, 1598-1564
49. Albucher JF, Ferrieres J, Ruidavets JB, Guirand-Chaumeil B, Perret BP, Chollet F: Serum lipids in
50. young patients with ischemic stroke: a case-control study. J Neurol Neurosurg Psychiatry 69, 2000, 29-33
51. Alter M, Lai SM, Friday G, Singh V, KumarVM, Sobel E: Stroke recurrence in diabetes. Does control of blood glucose reduce risk? Stroke 28, 1997, 1153-1157

52. Ambrosini E, Bacchellis S: Clinical approach to the hypertensive patient. New guidelines. Ann Ital Med Int 13, 1998,30-36
53. Arboix A, Garcia EL, Masson B, Olivers M, Gomes E: Predictive factors of early seizures after acute cerebrovascular disease. Stroke 28, 1997, 1590-1594
54. Arnold M, Sturzenegger M, Schaffler L, Seiler RW: Continuous intraoperative monitoring of middle cerebral artery blood flow velocities and electroencephalography during carotid endarterectomy. A comparison of two methods to detect cerebral ischemia. Stroke 28, 1997, 1345-1350
55. Aronov WS, Ahn C, Gutstein H: Risk factors for new atherothrombotic brain infarction in 664 older men and 1 448 women. Am J Cardiol 77, 1996, 1381-1383
56. Asokan G, Pareja J, Niedermeyer E: Temporal minor slow and sharp EEG activity and cerebrovascular disorder. Clin Electroencephalogr 18,1987,201-210
57. AuIIS, LaIouschek W, Schnider P, UhI F, ZeiIer K: DynamicChamges of plasma lipids and lipoproteins in patients after transient iaschemic attack or minor stroke. Am J Med 101, 1996, 291-298
58. Balkau B, Shipley M, Jarrett RJ, Pyorala K,
59. Pyorala M, Forhan A, Eschwede E: High blood glucose concentration is a risk factor for mortality in middle-aged nondiabetic men. 20-year follow-up in the Whitehall Study, and the Helsinki Policeman Study. Diabetes care 21, 1998, 360-367
60. Balotta E, Dagiau G, Saladini M, Bottio T, Abbruzzese E, Meneghretti G, Guera M: Results of electroencephalographic monitoring during 369 consecutive carotid revascularizations. Eur Neurol 37,1997,43-47
61. Banerjee R, Nageswari K, Puniyani RR: Association of hemorheological parameters and risk of stroke in hypertensives of Indian origin. Clin Exp Hypertens 22, 2000, 687-694
62. Barkis G: Joint National Committee on prevention, Detaction, Evaluation and treatment of High Blood Pressure. The Sixth Report of the Joint National Committee on Prevention, Detection, Evaluation and treatment of High Blood Pressure. Arch Intern Med 157, 1997, 2431-2446
63. Beaumanoir A, Andre-Obadia N, Nahory A, Zebri 0: Special types of periodic lateralized epileptiform discharges associated with confusional state in cerebral circulation insufficiency. Electroencephalogr Clin Neurophysiol 99, 1996, 287-292
64. Beckett N, Nunes M, Bulpitt C: Is it advantageous to lower cholesterol in the elderly hypertensive? Cardiovasc Drugs Ther 14, 2000, 397-405
65. Beks PH, Mackaay AJ, deVries H, de Neeling JH, Heine RL: Carotid artery stenosis is related to blood glucose level in an elderly Caucasian Population: the Hoorn Study. Diabetologia 40, 1997,290-298
66. Benjamin EJ, D'Agostino RB, Belanger AJ, Wolf PA, Levy D: Left arterial size and the risk of stroke and death. The Framingam Heart Study. Cirulation 92, 1995, 835-841

67. Berger K, Schulte H, Strogbauer F, Assamann G: Incidence and risk factors for stroke in an occupational cohort: the PROCAM study. Prospective Cardiovascular Muenster Study. Stroke 29, 1998, 1562-1566
68. Beser E, Bay tan SH, Akkoyunlu D, Gul M: Cigarette smoking, eating behavior, blood haematocrit level and body mass index. Ethiop Med J 33, 1995, 155-162
69. Bikkina M, Levy D, Evans JC, Larson MG, Banjamin EJ, Wolf PA, Castelli WP: Left ventricular mass and risk of stroke in the elderly cohort. The Framingam Heart Study. JAMA 272, 1994, 71-72
70. Bilora F, Vigna GB, Saccaro G, Pastorello MP, Polato G, Mainfredini C, Chiesa M, Barbara A, Vettore G, San Lorenzo L: Short term changes in risk factors of cerebrovascular diseases. Miverva Med 87,1996,439-448
71. Binnie CD, Prior PF: Electroencephalography. J Neurol Neurosurg Psychiatr 57, 1994, 1308-1319
72. Bodo M, Thuroczy G, Nagy I, Peredi J, Sipos K, Harcos P, Nagy Z, Voros J, Zoltay L, Ozsvald L: A complex cerebrovascular screening system (CEREBRUS). Med Prog Technol 21, 1885, 53-66
73. Bolinder J, Noren A, de Faire U, Wahren J: Smokeless tobacco use and atherosclerosis: an ultrasonographic investigation of carotid intima media thickness in healthy middle-aged men.
74. Atherosclerosis 132, 1997, 95-103
75. Bradley KA, Badrinath S, Bush K, Boyd-Wickizer B: Medical risk for womwn who drink alcohol. J Gen Intern Med 13, 1998,627639
76. Branin M, Badrinath S, Bush K, Boyd-Wickizer B: Medical rsk for women who drink alcohol. J Gen Intern Med 13, 1998,627-639
77. Brown R, Whisnant J, Sicks J, O'Fallon W, Wiebers D: Stroke incidence, prevalence and survival. Secular trends in Rochester, Minnesota, through 1989. Stroke 27, 1996, 373-380
78. Busser MG, Kittner SJ: Oral contraceptives and stroke. Cephalgia 20,2000,183-189
79. Caicoya M, Rodriguez T, Corrales C, Cuello R, Lasheras C: Alcohol and stroke: a community case-control study in Asturias, Spain. J Clin Epidemiol 52, 1999, 677-684
80. Campbell NR, Ashley J, Carruthers SG, Lacourciaere Y, Mc Kay OW: Lifestyle modifications to prevent and control hypertension. 3. Recommentation of alcohol consumption. Canadian Hypertension Society, Canadian Coalition for High Blood Pressure Prevention and Control, laboratory Center for Disease Control at Health Canada, Hearth and Stroke Foundation of Canada. CMAJ 160, 1999, 13-20
81. Carole L, Hole D, Smith G: Risk factors and 20-year Stroke Mortality in Men and Women in the Scotland. Stroke 30, 1999, 19992007
82. Catalano M, Perilli E, Carzaniga G, Colombo F, Carotta M, Andreoni S: Lp(a) in hypertensive patients. J Hum Hypertens 12, 199B! 83-89 .
83. Chambless LE, Shahar E, Sharett AR, Heiss G, Wijberg L, Paton CC, Sorlie P, Toole JF:

84. Association of transient ischemic attack (stroke symptoms assessed by standardized questionnaire and algorithm with cerebrovascular risk factor and carotid artery wall thickness). The ARIC study 1987-1989. Am J Epidemiol144, 1996,857-866
85. Chang CL, Donaghy M, Poulter N: Migraine and stroke in young women: case-control study. The World Health Organization Collaborative Study of Cerebrovascular Disease and Steroid Hormone Contraception. BJM 318, 1999, 13-18
86. Chaturvedi S, Yoom BW, Sharpe B, Eliasziw M, Fox A, Hachinski VC, Bartnett HJM: Clinical and angiographic outcome of medically treated severe carotid stenosis. Neurology 44, 1994,271
87. Chen WH, Chang YY, Chou MS, Lui JS: The lipoprotein profile of young adults with cerebral atherosclerosis. Southeast Asian J Trop Med Public Health 27, 1996, 178-183
88. Cheng SW, Wu LL, Lau H, Ting AC, Wong J: Prevalence of significant carotid stenosis in Chinese patients witj peripheral and coronary disease. Aust N, Surg 69, 1999,44-47
89. Chimowitz MI, Weiss DG, Cohen SL, Starling MR, Hobson RW: 2nd Cardiac prognosis of patients with carotid stenosis and no history of coronary artery disease. Veterans Affairs Cooperative Study Group 167. Stroke 25, 1994,759-765
90. Chimowitz MI, Poole RM, Starling MR, Schwaiger M, Gross MD: Frequency and severity of asymptomatic coronary disease in patients with different causes of stroke. Stroke 28, 1997,941-945 85. Chlumsky J, Charvat J: Echocardiography of carotid arteries in diabetics with cererovascular
91. stroke. Vnitr Lek 46, 2000, 848-850
92. Claeroux J, Feldman RD, Petrella BJ: Lifestyle modifications to prevent and control hypertension 4. Recommentation on physical exercise training. Canadian Hypertension Society, Canadian Coalition for High Blood- Pressure Prevention and Control, Laboratory Centre for Disease Control at Health Canada, Haerth and Stroke Foundation of Canada. CMAJ 160, 1999, 21-28
93. Cognazzo A, Grasso E, Gerbino-Promis PC, Zagnoni P: Frequency of risk factors in cerebrovascular disease and their effect on the course and outcome. Study on 423 hospitalized patients. Minerva Med 72, 1981, 2929-2934
94. Cohen SN, Hobson RW, Weiss DG, Chimowitz M: Death associated with asymptomatic carotid artery stenosis: Long term clinical evaluation. J Vasc Surg 18, 1993, 1002-1011
95. Cooper R, Cutler J, Desnigne-Nickens P, Fortmann SP, Friedman L, Havlic R, Hogelin G, Marler J, Mc Govern P, Morosco G, Mosca L, Pearson T, Samler J, Stryer D, Thom T: Trends and disparities in coronary hearth disease, stroke, and other cardiovascular diseases in the United States: finding of the national conference on cardiovascular disease prevention. Circulation 102, 2000, 3137-3147
96. Countinho M, Gerstein HC, Wang Y, Ysuf S: The relationship between glucose and incident cardiovascular events. A metaregression analysis of published data

from 20 studies of 95783 individuals for 124 years. Diabetes care 22, 1999, 233-240
97. Crouse JR, Goldbourt U, Evans G, Pnsky J,
98. Sharett AR, Sorlie P, Riley W, Heiss G: Risk factors and segment-specific carotid arterial enlargement in the Atherosclerosis Risk in Communities (ARIC) cohort. Stroke 27, 1996, 69-75
99. Curb JD, Abbot RD, Mac Lean CJ, Rodrigez BL, Burchfiel CM, Sharp OS, Ross GW, Yano K: Age-related changes in stroke risk in men hypertension and normal blood pressure. Stroke 27, 1996, 819-824
100. Currie CJ, Morgan CL, Gill L, Stott NC, Peters JP: Epidemiology and costs of acute hospital care for cerebrovascular disease in diabetic and nondiabetic population. Stroke 28, 1997, 1142-1146
101. D'Onofrio F, Salvia S, Petretta V, Bonavita V, Rodrigez G, Tedeschi G: Quantified EEG in normal aging and dementias. Acta Neurol Scand 93, 1996, 336-345
102. Davis BR, Vogt T, Frost PH, Burlando A, Cohen J, Wilson A, Brass LM, Frishman W, Price T, Stamler J: Risk facor for stroke and type of stroke in persons with isolated systolic hypertension. Systolic Hypertension in the Elderly Program Cooperative Research Group. Strok- 29. 1998, 1333-1340
103. Ue Lorirnier AA. Alcohoi, wine and heaith. Am J SUrg 180, 2000, 357-361
104. Donnan PT, Leese GP, Morris AD: Hospitalizations for people with type 1 and type 2 diabetes compared with the nondiabetic population of Tayside, Scotland: a retrospective cohort study of resource use. Diabetes care 23,2000, 1774-1779
105. Du X, Mc Namee R, Cruickshank K: Stroke risk from multiple risk factors combined with
106. hypertension: a primary care based case-control study in a defined population of northwest England. Ann Epidemiol10, 2000, 380-388
107. Dyker AG, Weir CJ, Lees KR: Influence of cholesterol on survival after stroke: retrospective study. BMJ 314,1997,1584-1588
108. Easton JD: Epidemiology of stroke recurrence. Cardiovasc Dis 7, 1997,2-4
109. EI Barghouti N, Elkeles R, Nicolaides A, Geroulakos G, Dhanjil S, Diamond J: The ultrasound evaluation of the carotid intima-media thickness and its relation to risk factors of atherosclerosis in nomal and diabetic population. Int Angiol16, 1997, 50-54
110. Elkeles RS, Diamond JR, EI-Bahghouti N, Dhanjil S, Nicolaides A, Geroulakos G, Renton S, Anyaoku V, Richmond W, Mather H, Sharp P: Relative fasting hypoinsulinemia and ultrasonically measured early arterial disease in type 2 diabetes. The SENDCAP Study Group, St Mary's Ealing, Northwick Park Diabetes Cardiovascular Disease Prevention Study. Diabet Med 13, 1996, 247-253
111. Ellekjaer EF, Wyller TB, Sverre JM, Holmen J: Lifestyle factors and risk of cerebral infarction. Stroke 23, 1998,829-834
112. Ellis MR, Franks PJ, Cumming R, Powell JT, Greenhalgen RM: Prevalence, progression and natural history of asymptomatic carotid stenosis: is there a place for carotid endarterectomy? Eur J Vasc Surg 6,1992, 172-177

113. Ezekowitz MD, James KE, Nazarian SM, Davenport J, Broderick JP, Gupta SR, Thadani V, Meyer ML, Bridgers SL: Silent cerebral
114. infarction in patients with in nonrheumatic atrial fibrillation. Circulation 92, 1995, 2178-2182
115. Falke P, Lingarde F, Stavenov L: Prognosis indicators for mortality in transient ischemic attacks and minor stroke. Acta Neurol Scand 90, 1994, 78-82
116. Fang XH, Kronmal RA, Li SC, Longstreth WT, Cheng XM, Wang WZ, Wu S, Du XL, Siccovick D: Prevention of stroke in urban China: a community interventional trial. Stroke 30, 1999, 495-501
117. Farley TM, Meirik D, Chang CL, Poulter NR: Combined oral contraceptives, smoking, and cardiovascular risk. J Epidemiol Community Health 52, 1998, 775-785
118. Farley TM, Meirik D, Cloons J: Cardivascular disease and combined oral contraceptives: reviewing the evidence and balancing the risks. Hum Reprod Update 5, 1999, 721-735
119. Feigin VL, Wiebers DO, Nikitin Y, O'Fallon WM, Whisnant JP: Risk factors for ischemic stroke in a Russian community: a population - based control study. Stroke 29, 1998, 34-39
120. Ferro JM, Crespo M: Prognosis after transient ischemic attacks and ischemic stroke in young adults. Stroke 25, 1994, 16111616
121. Florkowski CM, Scott RS, Moir CL, Graham PJ: Lipid but not glycaemic parameters predict total mortality from type 2 diabetes mellitus in Canterbury, New Zealand. Diabet Med 15, 1998,386392
122. Fonseca T, Cortes P, Monteiro J, Salgado V, Ferro AS, Noguera JB, Da Costa IN: Acute cerebrovascular disorder and arterial hypertension.
123. Prospective study with 248 patients. Rev Port Cardiol 15, 1996, 565-573
124. Franklin SS, Sutton-Tyrell K, Belle SH, Weber MA, Kuller LH: The importance of pulsative components of hypertension in predicting carotid stenosis in older adults. J Hypertens 15, 1997, 11431150
125. Frenandez-Bouzas A, Harmony T, Fernandez T, Silva-Pereyra J, Valdes P, Bosch J, Aubert E, Casian G, Otero Ojeda G, Ricardo J, Hernandez-Ballesteros A, Santiago E: Sources of abnormal EEG activity in brain infarction. Electroencephalogr 31, 2000, 165-169
126. Frimm CD, Trezza B, Gruppi C, Medeiros C, Curi M, Krieger E: Left ventricular hypertrophy predict outcome of hypertension regardless of the type of ventricular arrhythmia present. J Him Hypertens 13, 1999,617-623
127. Fulesdi B, Limburg M, Bereczki D, Michels RP, Neuwirth G, Legemate D, Valiakovics A, Csiba L: Impairment of cerebrovascular reactivity in long-term type 1 diabetes. Diabetes 46, 1997, 1840-1845
128. Gariballa SE: Nutritional factors in stroke. Br J Nutt 84, 2000, 5-17
129. Gervaise N, Garrigue MA, Lasfargues G, Lecomte P: Triglicerides, apo C_3 and cardiovascular risk in type II diabetes. Diabetologia 43, 2000, 703 -798
130. Gillum RF, Sempos Ch T: The end of the long-term decline in the stroke mortality in the United States? Stroke 28, 19997, 1527-1529

131. Giroud M, Creisson E, Fayolle H, Andre N, Becker F, Martin D, Dumas R: Risk factors for
132. primary cerebral hemorrhage a population-based study - the Registry of Dijon. Neuroepidemiology 14, 1995,20-26
133. Godsland IF, Winkler U, Lidegraard D, Crooc D: Occlusive vascular disease in oral contraceptive users. Epidemiology, pathology and mechanisms. Drugs 60, 2000, 721-869
134. Goff DC, D'Agostino RB, Haffner SM, Saad MF, Wagenknecht LE: Lipoprotein concentrations and carotid atherosclerosis by diabetes status: results from the Insulin Resistence Atherosclerosis Study. Diabetes care 23,2000, 1006-1011
135. Gottdiner JS, Arnold AM, Aurigemma GP, Polak JF, Tracy RP, Kitzman OW, Gardin JM, Rutledge JE, Boineau RC: Predictors of congestive heart failure in the elderly: the Cardivascular Heart Study. J Am Coli Cardiol 35, 2000, 1628-1637
136. Grobbee DE, Koudstaal PJ, Bots ML, Amaducchi LA, Elwood PC, Ferro J, Frei de Cocalves A, Kruger D, Inzitari D, Nikitin Y, Salonen JT, Sivenius J, Scheuermann W, Theile OS, Trichopulos' JT: Incidence and risk factors of ischemic and hemorrhadic stroke in Europe. EUROSTROKE: collaborative study among research centers in Europe: rationale and design. Neuroepidemiol 15, 1996, 291-300
137. Gronholdth ML, Nordestgaard BG, Nielsen TG, Sillesen H: Echolucent carotid artery plaques are associated with elevated levels of fasting and postprandial triglyceride-rich lipoproteins. Stroke 27, 1996, 2166-2172
138. Gronholdth ML, Nordestgaard BG, Wiebe BM, Wilhjelm JE, Sillesen H: Echolucency of computerized ultrasound images of carotid
139. atherosclerosis plaques are associated with increased levels of triglyceride-rich lipoproteins as well as increased plaque lipid content. Circulation 97, 1998, 34-40
140. Guo Z, Vitanen M, fratiglioni L, Winblad B: Blood pressure and dementia in the elderly: epidemiologic perspectives. Biomed Pharmacother 51, 1997, 68-73
141. Hachinski V, Graffagnino C, Beaudry M, Donner A, Spence JD, Doig G, Wolf BM: Lipids and stroke: a paradox resolved. Arch Neurol 53, 1996, 303-308
142. Hadjiev D, Manchev I, Tsoneva-Pencheva L: Epidemiological investigation of the early forms of cerebrovascular disease-Ia-tent insufficiency and transient ischemic attacks. In: *Modern trends in neurological emergencies.* Prague, April 18th - 22nd, 1988, 148
143. Hadjiev D: Epidemiology of stroke. In: Bergen DC, Chopra JS, Silberberg D, Barac B, Lechner H (eds.) *Progress in Neurology-II.* BI Churchill Livingston Pvt Ltd, New Delphi, 1998, pp. 66-71
144. Haheim LL, Holme I, Hjermann I, Leren P: Risk of fatal stroke according to blood pressure level: an 18-year follow-up the Oslo Study. J Hypertension 13, 1995, 909-913
145. Haheim LL, Holme I, Hjermann I, Leren P: Smoking abits and risk of fatal stroke: 18 years follow-up of the Oslo Study. J Epidemiol Community Health 50, 1996, 612-624

146. Hajat C, Dundas R, Steward JA, Lawrence E, Rudd AG, Howard R, Wolfe CD: Cerebrovascular risk factors and stroke subtypes: Differences between ethnic groups. Stroke 32, 2001, 37-42
147. Hannaford PC, Croft PR, Kay CR: Oral contraception and stroke. Evidence from the Royal College of General Practioners'. Oral contraception study. Stroke 25,1994, 935-942
148. Hart CL, Smith GO, Hole OJ, Hawthorne VM: Alcohol consumption and mortality from all causes, coronary heart and stroke: results from a prospective cohort study of Scottish men with 21 years of follow-up. BMJ 318, 1999, 1725-1729
149. Hart L, Hole OJ, Smith GO: Cmparison of risk factors for stroke incidence and stroke mortality in 20 years of follow-up in men and women in the Renfrew. Paisley Study in Scotland. Stroke 31, 2000, 1893-1896
150. He J, klad J, Wu Z, Whelton PK: Stroke in the People's Republic China. Meta-analysis of the hypertension and risk of stroke. Stroke 26, 1995, 2228-2232
151. Heinemann LA: Emerging evidence on oral contraceptives and arterial disease. Contraception 62, 2000, 295-365
152. Heinemann LA, Lewis MA, Thorogood M, Spitzer WO, Guggnmoos-Holzmann I, Bruppacher R: Case-control study of oral contraceptives and risk of thromboembolic stroke: results from International Study on Oral contraceptives and Health of Young Women. BMJ 315,1997,1502-1504
153. Heinemann LA, Lewis MA, Spitzer WO, Thorogood M, Guggnmoos-Holzmann I, Bruppacher R: Thromboembolic stroke in young women. An European case-control study on oral contraceptives. Transnational Research Group on Oral contraceptives and the Health of Young
154. Women. Contraception 57, 1998, 29-37
155. Hempel HD, Schmidt RM: Frequency pattern of alpha waves in the early stages of cerebrovascular circulation disorders. Psychiatr Neurol Med Psychol Leipz 27, 1975, 348-351
156. Hennekens CH: Lessons from hypertension trials. Am J Med 104, 1998, 50-53
157. Hobson RW, Weisss DG, Fields WS, Goldstone J, Moore WS, Towne J8, Wright G8 and the Vterans Affair Cooperative Stufy Group: Efficacy of carotid endarterectomy for asymptomatic carotid stenosis. N Engl J Med 328, 1993, 221-227
158. Hodis HN, Mack WJ, Dunn M, Liu C, Selzer RH, Krauss RM: Intermediate-density lipoprotein and progression of carotid arterial wall intima-media thickness. Circulation 95, 1997, 2022-2026
159. Honczarenko K, Torbus-Lisiecka 8, Osuch Z, Nocon 0, Nowacki P, Potemkowski A, Narolewska A: Fibrinogen and lipids: associated risk factors for ischemic cerebral strike. Neurol Neurochir Pol 33, 1999, 557-656
160. Hougaku H, Matsumoto M, Handa H, Maeda H, Iton T, Tsukamoto Y, Kamada T: Asymptomatic carotid lesions and silent cerebral infarction. Stroke 25, 1994, 566-570

161. House AK, 8ell R, House J, Mastaglia F, Kumar A, D'Antuono M: Asymptomatic carotid artery stenosis associated with peripheral vascular disease: a prospective study. Cardiovasc Surg 7, 1999, 44-49
162. Howard G, Wagenknecht LE, cai J, Cooper L, Kraut MA, Toole JF: Cigarette smoking and other risk factors for silent cerebral infarction in the general population. Stroke 29, 1998, 913-917
163. Hu HH, Tzeng SS: Ischemic stroke in Taiwan. J Formosan Med Assoc 93, 1994,6-12
164. Hulte J, Wikstrand J, Emanuelsson H, Wiklung D, de Feyter PJ, Wenderlhag I: Atherosclerotic changes in the carotid artery bulb as measured by 8-mode ultrasound are associated with the extent of coronary atherosclerosis. Stroke 28, 1997, 1189-1194
165. Inui K, Sannan H, Ota H, Uji Y, Nomura S, Kaige H, Kitayama I, Nomra J: EEG finding in diabetic patients with and without retinipathy. Acta Neurol Scand 97, 1998, 107-109
166. Iribarren C, Jacobs DR, Sadler M, Claxton AJ, Sydney S: Low total serum cholesterol and intracerebral hemorrhagic stroke is the association confined to elderly men? The Keiser Permanente Medical Care Program. Stroke 27, 1996, 1993-1998
167. Luama A, Inouye T, Ukai S, Shiminosaki K: Spindle activity in the walking EEG in older adults. Clin Electroencephalogr 23, 1992, 137-141
168. Jacobs DR: The relationship between cholesterol and stroke. Health Report 6,1994,87-93
169. Jedrzeiowska H, Lysakowska-Sernicka K, Krolikiewicz-Sciborowska H Szirkowiec-Gmurczyk W: Arterial hypertension, diabetes and cardiac arrhythmias as risk factor in reversible and completed ischemic stroke. Neurol Neurochir Pol 30, 1996, 559-570
170. Johnson SC, Colford JM, Gress DR: Oral contraceptives and risk of subarachnoid hemorrhage: a meta-analysis. Neurology 51, 1998, 411-418
171. Jorgensen HS, Nakayama H, Raaschou HO,
172. Olsen TS: Stroke in patients with diabetes. The Copenhagen Stroke Study. Stroke 25, 1994, 1997-1984
173. Jorgensen HS, Nakayama H, Reith J, Raaschou HO, Olsen TS: Acute stroke with atrial fibrillation. The Copenhagen Stroke Study. Stroke 27, 1996, 1765-1769
174. Jorgensen HS, Nakayama H, Reith J, Raaschou HO, Olsen TS: stroke reccurence: predictors, severity and prognosis. Copenhagen Stroke Study. Neurology 48, 1997, 891-895
175. Jousilahti P, Rastenyte 0, Tuomilehto J, Sarti C, Variainen E: Parental history of cardiovascular disease and risk of stroke. A prospective follow-up of 14371 middle-aged men and women in Finland. Stroke 28,1997,1361-1366
176. Jover-Saenz A, Porcel-Perez JM, Vives-Soto M, Rubio-Caballero M: Epidemiology of acute cerebrovascular disease in Ll eida from 1996 to 1997. Predictive factors of mortality at short and medium term. Rev Neurol 28, 1999, 941-948

177. Kaarisalo MM, Immonen-Raiha P, Marttila RL, Lehtonen A, Salomaa V, Sarti C, Sivenius J, Torppa J, Tuomilehto J: Atrial fibrillation in older stroke patients: association with reccurence and mortality after first ischemic stroke. J AM Geriatr Soc 45, 1997, 12271231
178. Kadojiyc D, Demarin V, Kadojiyc M, Mihaljeviyc I, Barac B: Influence of prolonged stress on risk factors for cerebrovascular disease. Coli Antropol 23, 1999,213-219
179. Kalra L, Perez I, Melbourn A: Stroke risk management: changes in mainstream practice. Stroke 29,2000, 165-169
180. Kameyama S, Tanimura K, Honda Y: Correlation between alpha wave patter of regional cerebral blood flow. No To Shinkei 36, 1984, 1229-1235
181. Kannel WB: Epidemiology of cerebrovascular Disease. In: RW Ross Russel (ed) *Cerebral arterial disease.* Churchill Livingston, Edinburgh, London, New York, 1997, pp. 1-23
182. Kaukura J, Turpeinen A, Uusitupa M, Niskanen L: Clustering of cardiovascular risk factors in type 2 diabetes mellitus: prognostic significance and tracking. Diabetes Obes Metab 3,2002, 17-23
183. Kiechl S, Willeit J, Rungger G, Egger G, Oberholenzer F, Bonora E: Alcohol consumption and atherosclerosis: what is the relation? Stroke 29, 1998, 900-907
184. Kilander L, Nyman H, Boberg M, Hansson L, Lithell H: Hypertension is related to cognitive impairment: a 20-year follow-up of 999 men. Hypertension 31, 1998, 780-786
185. Kocemba J, Kawecka-Jaszcz K, Grylewska B, Grodzicki T: Isolated systolic hypertension: pathophysiology, consequences and therapeutic benefits. J Hum Hypertens 12, 1998, 621-626
186. Koefoed BG, Gullov AL, Petersen P: Atrial fibrillation and apoplexy- risk and Nord Med 111, 1996, 171-175
187. Korpelainen JT, Sotaniemi KA, Huikuri HV, Myllya VV: Abnormal heart rate variability as a manifestation of autonomic dysfunction in hemispheric brain infarction. Stroke 27, 1996, 2059-2063
188. Kowal P: Continued study of factors influencing the amount of shear wall stress in the acute phase
189. of ischemic stroke. Przeglad Lakarski52, 1995, 382-384
190. Kubota K, Tamura K, Take H, Kurabayashi H, Shirakura T: Acute myocardial infarction Kusatsu - spa. Nippon Ronnen Igakkai Zasshi34, 1997, 23-29
191. Lado-Lado FL, Sanches-Leira J, Alende-Sixto R, Calvo-Gomez C, Martinez-Vazquez JM, Barrio-Gomez E: Cerebrovascular disease and assotiated risk factors. Ann Med Intern 13, 1996, 527-530
192. Landray MJ, Sagar G, Muskin J, Murray S, Holder RL, Lip GY: Association of atherogenic low-density lipoprotein subfractions with carotid atherosclerosis. QLM 91, 1998, 345-351
193. Lechner H, Ott E, Fazekas F: Prevention of stroke: current trends and knowledge. In: Lechner E, Mayer JS, OU E (eds.) Cerebrovascular disease: Research and

clinical management. Elsevier, Amsterdam, New York, Oxford, 1986, pp. 219-229
194. Lechner H, Hadjiev D: Epidemiology of cerebrovascular risk factors in Southeast Europe. 11th Thessaloniki Conference. Thessaloniki, Abstract volume, sept. 1996, 25-28
195. Lechner H, Hadjiev D: Comparative epidemiological study on cerebrovascular risk factors among Australian and Bulgarian population. Neurol Psychiatry Brain Res 6, 1998, 141-146
196. Lechner H, Hadjiev D, Schmidt GL: Basis elements for developing a stroke reduction program in countries with high stroke incidence and a health act for prevention. In The 20th Salzburg Conferenceq Nov 3-6, 1999, Abstracts,
197. p. 15
198. Ledegaard D: Smoking and use of oral contraceptives: impact on thrombotic disease. Am J Obstet Gynecol180, 1999,53575363
199. Leira R: Migraine due to infarct. Neurologia 5, 1997, 16-23 184. Leonardt G, Diener HC: Epidemiology and risk factors in stroke. Ther Umsch 53, 1996, 512-518
200. Leppala JM, Paunio M, Virtamo J, Fogelholm R, Albanes D, Taylor PR, Heinonen OP: Alcohol consumption and stroke incidence in male smokers. Circulation 14, 1999a, 1209-1214
201. Leppala JM, Virtamo J, Fogelholm R, Albanes D, Heinonen OP: Different risk factors dofferent stroke subtypes: association of blood pressure, cholesterol, and antioxidants. Stroke 30, 1999b, 2535-2540
202. Lestro-Henriques I, Bogouslavsky L, van Malle G: Predictors of strike pattern in hypertensive patients. J Neurol Sci 144, 1996, 142-146
203. Levine SR, Fagan SC, Pessin MS, Silberglet R, Floberg J, Selva JF, Vogel CM, Welch KM: Accelerated intracranial occlusive disease oral contraceptives, and cigarette use. Neurology 41, 1991, 1893-1901
204. Udegaard D, Kreiner S: Cerebral thrombosis and oral contraceptives. A case-control study. Contraception 57, 1998, 303-314
205. Un HJ, Wolf PA, Kelley-Hayes M, Beiser AS, Kase CS, Benjamin EJ, D'Agostino RB: Stroke severity in atrial fibrillation. The Framingam Study. Stroke 27, 1996, 1760-1754
206. Udenstrom E, Boysen G, Nyboe J: Infuence of systolic and diastolic blood pressure on stroke risk:
207. a prospective observational study. Am J Epidemiol142, 1995, 1279-1290
208. Logar C, Schmidt R, Freidl W, Reinhart B, Scala M, Lechner H: EEG mapping in middle aged normal volunteers: the impact of cerebrovascular risk factors. Brain Topogr 6, 1993, 111-115
209. Loungstreth WT, Shemanski L, Lefkowitz OM, O'Leary DH, Polak JF, Wolfson SC: Asymptomatic internal carotid artery stenosis defined by ultrasound and the risk of subsequent stroke in the elderly. The Cardiovascular Health Study. Stroke 29, 1998,2371-2376

210. Lowe GO, Lee AJ, Rumley A, Price JF, Fowkers FG: Blood viscosity and risk of cardiovascular events the Edinburgh Artery Study. Br J Haemtol 96,1997,168-173
211. Mac Mahon S, Peto R, Culter J, Collins R, Sorlie P, Neaton J, Abbott R, Godwin J, Dyer A, Stamler J: Blood pressure, stroke, and coronary heart disease, part 1: prolonged differences in blood pressure: prospective observational studies corrected regression dilution bias. Lancet 335, 1990,756-774
212. Mackey AE, Abramowitz M, Langois Y, Battista R, Simard O, Bourque F, Leclerc I, Cote R: Outcome of asymptomatic patients wioth carotid disease. Neurology 48, 1997, 896-903
213. Malacher AM, Schultman J, Epstein LA, Thun MJ, Mowery P, Pierce B, Escobedo L, Giovino GA: Methodological issues in estimating smoking - attributive mortality in the United States. Am J Epidemiol 152, 2000, 573-584
214. Manaffrey KV, Harrington RA, Simoons ML, Granger CB, Graffagnino C, Alberts MJ,
215. Laskowitz OT, Miller JM, Sloan MA, Berdan LG, Mac Aulay CM, Uncoff AM, Deckers J, Topol EJ, Califf RM: Stroke in patients with acute coronary syndromes: incidence and outcomes in the platelet glycoprotein Ilb/lla in instable angina. Receptor suppression using intergilin therapy (PURSUIT) trial. The PURSUIT Investigators. Circulation 99, 1999,2371-2377
216. Mankowsky BN, Metzger BE, Molitch ME, Biller J: Cerebrovascular disorders in patients with diabetes mellitus. J Diabetes Complications 10, 1996, 228-242
217. Mannami T, Konishi M, Baba S, Nishi N, Terao A: Prevalence of asymptomatic carotid atherosclerosis lesions detected by high resolution ultrasonography and its relation to cardiovascular risk factors in the general population of a Japanese city: the Suita Study. Stroke 28, 1997, 518-525
218. Mannami T, Baba S, Ogata J: Strong and significant relationship between aggregation of carotid atherosclerosis in the general population of a Japanese city: the Suita Study. Arch Intern Med 160, 2000, 2297-2303
219. Manolio TA, Kronmal RA, Burke GL, O'Leary DH, Price TR: Short-term predictors of incident stroke in older adults. The Cardio-vascular Health Study. Strike 27, 1996, 1479-1486
220. Mansour MA, Uttooy FN, Watson WC, Blumofe KA, Heilizer T J, Steffen GF, Chmura C, Kang SS, Labropoulos N, Greisler HP, Fischer SG, Baker WH: Outcome of moderate carotid artery stenosis in patients who are asymptomatic. J Vasc Surg 29, 1999, 217-225
221. Marand van de Mheen PJ, Gunning-Schepers LJ:
222. Variation between studies in report relative risk associated with hypertension: time trends and other explanatory variables. Am J Public Health 88, 1998, 618-622
223. Marini C, Totaro R, Carolei A: Long-term Prognosis of Gerebrallschemia in Young Adults. Stroke 30, 1999,2320-2325

224. Mast H, Koenneckle HC, Hartmann A, Stapf C, Marx P: Association of hypertension and diabetes mellitus with microangiopathic cerebral infarct patterns. Nervenarzt 68,1997,129134
225. Mast H, Thompson JL, Un IF, Hofmeister C, Hartmann A, Marx P, Mohr JP, Sacco RL: Cigarette smoking as a determinant of high-grade carotid artery stenosis in Hispanicq black, and white patients with stroke or transient ischemic attack. Stroke 29, 1998, 918-1112
226. Maynard SO, Hudges JR: A distinctive entity: burst of rhythmical temporal theta. Clin Electroencephalogr 15, 1984, 145-150
227. Medical Research Council Working Party. MRS Trial of treatment of mild hypertension: Principal results. BMJ 291, 1985,97-104
228. Megnien JL, Denarie N, Cocaul M"Simon A, Levenson J: Predictive value ofwist-to-hip ratio on cardiovascular risk events. Int JObes Relat Metab Disor 23, 1999, 90-97
229. Meister KA, Whelan EM, Kava R: The health effects of moderate alcohol intake in humans: an epidemiological review. Crit Clin Lab Sci 37, 2000, 261-296
230. Menotti A, Jacobs D, Blackburn H, Kromhout, Nissinen A, Nedelkovic S, Buzina RI, Seccareccia F, Giampaoli S, Donatas A, Aravanis CH,
231. Toshima H: Twenty-five year prediction of stroke death in the Seven Countries Study. The role of the blood pressure and its changes. Stroke 27, 1996, 381-387
232. Merikangas KR, Fenton BT, Cheng SH, Stolar MJ, Risch N: Association between migraine and stroke in a large-scale epidemiological study of the United States. Arch Neurol 54, 1997,362-368
233. Mhurchu CN, Anderson C, Jamrozik K, Hankey G, Dunbabin D: Australasian Cooperative Research on Subarachnoid Hemorrhage Study (ACROSS) Group. Hormonal factors and risk of aneurismal subarachnoid hemorrhage: an Internation population based case-control study. Stroke 32,2000,606-612
234. Misumi I, Kimura Y, Hokamure Y, Honda Y, Misumi K, Yamabe H, Fukushima T, Emura Y, Mauyama H, Ohsawa E: Acute left ventricular thrombosis in patients with cerebral hemorrhage. Intern Med 36, 1997, 92-96
235. Modredo-Pardo PJ, Labrador-Fuster T, Torres-Nuez J: Silent brain infarctions in patients with coronary heart disease. A Spanish population survey. J Neurol 245, 1998,93-97
236. Molnar M, Gacs G, Ujvari G, Skinner JE, Karmos G: Dimensional complexity of the EEG in the subcoritical stroke - a case study. Int J Psychophysiol 25, 1997, 193-199
237. Mooe T, Eriksson P, Stegmeyr B: Ischemic stroke after aĸute mypcardial infarction. A population-based study. Stroke 28, 1997 762-767
238. Mortando RM: Lipid level. Applying the Second National Cholesterol Education Program Report to Geriatric Medicine. Geroatrics 55,2000,48-53
239. Mortel KF, Meyer JS: Prospective study of vascular events and cerebral perfusional changes following transient ischemic attacks. Angiology 47, 1996,215-224

240. Muluk SC, Muluk VS, Sugimoto H, Rhee RY, Trachtenberg J, Steed DL, Jarett F, Webster MW, Makaroun MS: Progression of asymptomatic carotid stenosis. A natural history study in 1004 patients. J Vasc Surg 29, 1999,208-216
241. Nagi M, Prefferkorn T, Haberl RL: Blood glucose and stroke. Nervenartz 70, 1999, 944-949
242. Naidoo B, Stevens W, Mc Pherson K: Modelling the short term consequences of smoking cessation rates for acute myocardial infarction and stroke. Tob Control 9,2000,397-400
243. Nakayama K, Ichinose M: Ischemic stroke in elderly patients with paroxysmal atrial fibrillation. Nippon Ronen Igakkai Zasshi 1996, 273-277
244. Nakayama T, Date C, Yokoyama T, Yoshiike N, Yamaguchi M, Tanaka H: A 15.5-year follow-up study of stroke in a Japanese provincial city. The Shibata Study. Stroke 28, 1997, 45-52
245. Narbone MC, Leggiadro N, La-Spina P, Rao R, Gruno R, Musolino R: Migraine stroke: a possible complication of both migraine with and without aura. Headache 36, 1996,481-483
246. Ni Mhurchu C, Rogers A, Mac Mahon S: The associations of diastolic blood pressure with the risk of stroke in Western and Eastern populations. Clin Exp Hypertens 21, 1999, 531-542
247. Nideremeyer E, Da Silva FL: *Electroencephalography*, 2nd ed, Urban and Schwarzenberg, Baltimore, 1987
248. Nielsen WB, Vestbo J, Jensen GB: Isolated systolic hypertension: a significant risk factor of cerebral apoplexy and acute myocardial infarction. A prospective population based study. UgerskrLaeger158,1996,3779-3783
249. Nishino M, Sueyoshi K, Yasuno M, Yamada Y, Abe H, Hori H, Kamada T: Risk factors for carotid atherosclerosis and silent cerebral infarction patient with coronary heart disease. Angiology 44, 1993, 432-440
250. Niskanen L, Turpeinen A, Penttila I, Usitupa MI: Hyperglycemia and compositional lipoprotein abnormalities as predictors of cardiovascular mortality in type 2 diabetes: a 15-year follow-up from time of dignosis. Diabetes care 21, 1998, 1861-1869
251. Njolstad I, Arnesen E, Lund-Larsen PG: Cardiovascular diseases and diabetes mellitus in different ethnic groups: the Finnmark study. Epidemiology 5, 1998, 550-556
252. Norris JW, Zhu CZ, Bornstein NM, Chambers BR: Vascular risk of asymptomatic carotid stenosis. Stroke 22, 1991, 1485-490
253. Numminen H, Syrjala M, Benthin G, Kaste M, Hillbom M: The effect of acute ingestion of a large dose of alcohol on the haemostatic system and its circadian variation. Stroke 31, 2000, 1269-1273
254. O'Leary DH, Anderson KM, Wolf PA, Evans JC, Poehlman HW: Cholesterol and carotid atherosclerosis in older persons: The Framingam Study. Ann Epidemiol 2, 1992, 147-153
255. Okin PM, Roman MJ, Devereux RB, Klingfield P: Association of carotid atherosclerosis with electrocardiographic myocardial ischemia and left
256. ventricular hypertrophy. Hypertension 28, 1996, 3-7

257. Orencia AJ, Daviglus ML, Dyer AR, Walch M, Greenland P, Stamler J: One-hour post load plasma glucose and risk of fatal coronary heart disease and stroke among nondiabetic men and women: the Chicago Heart Association Detection Project in Industry (CHA) Study. Clin Epidemiol 50, 1997, 1369-1376
258. Otsuka K, Cornelissen G, Halberg F, Oehlerts G: Extensive circadian amplitude of blood pressure increases risk of ischemic stroke and nephropathy. J Med Eng Technol 21, 1997, 23-30
259. Ozawa H, Aono H, Saito I, Ikebe T: Atherosclerois and clinical examination: epidemiology of stroke and ischemic heart disease. Rinsho Byori 44, 1996, 1015-1026
260. Paffenbarger RS, Williams JL: Chronic disease in former college students. Early precursors of fatal stroke. Am J Public Health 57, 1967, 1290-1299
261. Paffenbarger RS, Williams JL: Chronic disease in former college students. Early precursors of fatal stroke. Am J Public Health 94, 1971, 524-530
262. Pan WH, Bai CH, Chen JR, Chiu HC: Associations between carotid atherosclerosis and high factor VIII activity, dyslipidemia and hypertension. Stroke 28, 1997, 88-94
263. Papadakis JA, Mikhaildis DP, Winder AF: Lipids and stroke: neglect of a useful preventive measure? Cardiovasc Res 40, 1998, 265-271
264. Parving HH: Diabetic hypertensive patients. Is this a group in need of particular care and attention? Diabetes Care 22, 1999, 76-79
265. Perron AD, Brandy WJ:
266. Electroencephalographic manifestations of CNS events. Am J Emerg Med 18, 2000, 715-720
267. Petrovitch H, Curb GO, Bloom-Marcus E: Isolated systolic hypertension and risk of stroke in Japanese-American men. Stroke 26, 1995, 25-29
268. Pohjasvaara T, Erkinjuntti T, Vataja R, Kaste M: Comparison of stroke features and disability in daily life in patients with ischemic stroke aged 55 to 71 to 85 years. Stroke 28, 1997, 729-739
269. Pop GA, Koudstaal PJ, Meeder HJ, Algra A, Van Latum JC, Van Gijn J: Predictive value of clinical history electroencephalogram in patients with transient ischemic attack or minor stroke for subsequent
270. cardial and cerebral ischemic events. The Dutch TIA Trial Study Group. Arch Neurol 51, 1994, 333-341
271. Postorino G, Altavilla R, Fantozii G, Provenzanno B, Capelli R, Forconi S: Is there a relationship between sex, age, Lp(a) blood levels, lipid values, and atherosclerotic carotid lesions? Mierva Med 87, 1996, 379-383
272. Pujia A, Rubba P, Spencer MP: Prevalence of extracranial carotid artery disease detectable by echo-Doppler in an elderly population. Stroke 23, 1992, 818-822
273. Qizilbash N: are risk factors for stroke and coronary disease the same? Curr Opin Lipidol 9, 1988, 325-358
274. Qureshi AI, Giles WS, Croft JB: Impaired glucose tolerance and the likelihood of nonfatal sroke and myocardial infarction: the Third National Health and Nurtition Examination Survey. Stroke 29, 1998, 1329-1332

275. Rasmussen BK: Migraine and tension - type headache in The general population: precipitationg factors, female hormones, sleep pattern and relation to life style. Pain 53, 1993,65-72
276. Resch KL, Ernst E: Rheologic risk factors of apoplexy. Versicherungsmedizin 42, 1990,103-106
277. Ricci S, Flamini FO, Celani MG, Marini M, Antonini D, Bartolini S, Ballatori E: Prevalence of internal carotid artery stenosis in subjects older than 49 years: A population study. Cerebrovasc Ois 1, 1991, 16-19
278. Rigaud AS, Seux ML, Staenssen JA, Birkenhager WH, Forette F: Cerebral complications of hypertension. J Hum Hypertens 14,2000,605-616
279. Ruff LK, Volmer T, Nowak D, Mayer A: The economic impact of smoking in Germany. Eur Respir J 16, 2000, 385-390
280. Ruivo A, Lopes M, Melo TR, Salgado AV, Olivera V, Canhao P, Pinto AN, Crespo M, Ferro JM: Carotid stenosis associated with artial fibrillation. Rev Neurol 24, 1996, 55-58
281. Sacco RL, Benjamin EJ, Broderick JP, Dyken M, Easton JD, Feinberg WM, Goldstein LW, Gorelick PB, Howard G, Kittner SJ, Manolio TA, Whisnant JP, Wolf PA: AHA Conference Proceeding. Risk factors. Stoke 28, 1997, 1507-1517
282. Sakamoto K, Saitoh S, Takagi S, Shimamoto K: Significance of accumulation of atherosclerosis risk factors in elderly people: from a study conducted in Tanno-Sobetsz. Nippon Ronen Igakkai Zasshi 35, 1998,382-388
283. Sankai T, Iso H, Shimamoto T, Kitamura A,
284. Naito Y, Stao S, Okamura T, Imano H, Iida M, Komachi Y: Prospective study on alcohol
285. intake and risk of subarachonoid hemorrhage among Japanese men and women. Alcohol Clin Res 24, 2000, 386-389
286. Santos-Lasaosa S, Lopez del Val J, Iniguez C, Ortells M, Escalza I, Navas I: Diabetes mellitus and stroke. Rev Neurol31, 2000, 14-16
287. Sato K, Kamiya S, Okawa M, Hozumi S, Hori H, Hishikawa Y: On the EEG component waves of multi-infarct dementia senilis. Int J Neurosci 86, 1996,95-109
288. Schleiffer T, Holken H, Brass H: Morbidity in 565 type 2 diabetic patients according to stage of nephropathy. J Diab Comlic 12, 1998, 103-109
289. Schradder J, Rothemeyer M, Luders S, Kollman K: Hypertension and stroke-rationale behinf the ACCESS trial. Acute Candesartan Cilecetil Evaluation in Stroke Survivors. Basis Res Card ion 93, 1998, 69-78
290. Sen S, Oppenheimer SM: Cardiac disorders and stroke. Curr Opin Neurol11, 1998, 51-56
291. Sesso HO, Stampfer MJ, Rosner B, Hannekens CH, Gaziano JM, Manson JE, Glynn RJ: Systolic and diastolic blood pressure, pulse pressure, and mean arterial pressure as predictors of cardiovascular disease risk in Men. Hypertension 36, 2000, 801-807

292. Sharma AK, Mehrotra TN, Goel VK, Mitra A, Sood K, Nath M: Clinical profile of stroke in relation to glycaemic status of patients. J Assoc Physician India 44, 1996, 19-21
293. Sharret AR, Sorlie PO, Chambless LE, Folsom AR, Hutchinson RG, Heiss G, Szklo M: Relative
294. importance of various risk factors for asymptomatic carotid atherosclerosis risk in communities study. Am J Epidemiol 49, 1999, 843-852
295. Shimamoto T, Iso H, Iida M, Komachi Y: Epidemiology of catdiovascular disease stroke epidemic in Japan. J Epidemiol 6, 1996,43-47
296. Shively BK, Geldand EA, Crawford MH: Regional left arterial during arterial fibrillation and flutter: determination and relation to stroke. J Am Coli Cardiol27, 1996, 1722-1729
297. Sich D, Saidi Y, Giral P, Lagrost L, Egloff M, Auer C, Gautier V, Turpin G, Beucler I: Hyperalphalipoproteinemia: characterization of cardioprotective profile associating increased high-density lipoprotein 2 levels and decreased hepatic lipase activity. Metabolism 47, 1998,965-973
298. Simons LA, Mc Callum J, Friedlander Y, Simons J: Risk factors for ischemic stroke: Oubbo Study of the elderly. Stroke 29, 1998, 1341-1346
299. Singh PN, Lindsted KO: Body mass and 26-year risk of mortality from specific disease among women who never smoked. Epidemiology 9,1998, 227-228
300. Siownik A, Zwolinska G, Tomik B, Wyrwicz-Petkow U, Szczudlik A: Prognostic significance of transient hyperglycemia in acute phase of ischemic stroke. Neurol Neurochir Pol 32, 1998,317- 329
301. Sochurkova D, Moreau T, Lemele M, Menassa M, Giroud M, Dumas R: Migraine history and migraine-induced stroke in the Dijon stroke registry. Neuroepidemiology 18, 1999,85-91
302. Somes GW, Pahor M, Shorr RI, Gusman WC, Applegate WB: The role of diastolic blood pressure when treating isolated systolic
303. hypertension. Arch Intern Med 27, 1999,2004-2009
304. Staessen JA, Thijs L, Fagard R, O'Brien ET, Clement OJ De Leeuw PW, Mancia G, Nachev C, Palatini P, Parati G, Tuomilehto J, Webster J: Predicting cardiovascular risk using conventional vs. ambulatory blood pressure in older patients with systolic hypertension. Systolic Hypertension in Europe Trial Investigators. JAMA 282, 1999, 539-546
305. Stegmayr B, Asplung K, Kuulasmaan K, Rajakangas A, Thorvaldsen P, Tuomilehto J: for yhe WHO MONICA Project, Stroke incidence and mortality correlated to stroke risk factors in the WHO MONICA Project. Stroke 28, 1997, 1367-1374
306. Steingrub JS, Mundt OJ: Blood glucose and neurologic outcome with global brain ischemia. Crit Care Med 24, 1996, 802-806
307. Stevens J, Tyroler HA, Cai J, Paton CC, Folsom AR, Tell GSm Schreiner PJ, Chambless LE: Body weight change and carotid artery wall thickness. The Atherosclerosis Risk in Communities (ARIC) Study. Am J Epidemiol 147, 1998, 563-573

308. Stoy NS: Stroke and cholesterol: "enigma variations"? J R Coli Physicians 31, 1997,521-526
309. Suter PM, Hasler E, Vetter W: Control of blood pressure: a key factor in prevention. Schweiz Rundsch Med Prax 87, 1998, 145-156
310. Suzuki A, Nishimura H, Yoshioka K, Iwase M, Yasui N, Hatazawa J, Kanno J: New display methods of combined topographic EEG and cerebral blood flow images in the evaluation of cerebral ischemia. Brain Topogr 8, 1996, 275-278
311. Teal PA, Norris JW: Medical consideration. In: HMJ Barnett, JP Mohr, BM Stein, FM Yatsu (eds.) *Stroke. Pathophysiology, Diagnosis and Management.* Third edition. Churchill Livingston, New York, 1998, pp. 1199-1209
312. Teno S, Uto Y, Nagashima H, Endoh Y, Iwamoto Y, Omori Y, Takizawa T: Association of postprandial hypertrigliceridemia and carotid intima-media thickness in patients with type 2 diabetes. Diabetes care 23,2000, 1401-1406
313. The SPAF III Writing Committee for the Stroke Prevention in Atrial Fibrillation Investigators: Patients with non-valvular atrial fibrillation at low risk of stroke during treatment with aspirin: Stroke Prevention in Atrial Fibrillation III Study. JAMA 279,1998,1273-1277
314. Thomas M, Olafsson B, Stegmayr B, Erikson P: Ischemic stroke impact of recent myocardial infarction. Stroke 33, 1999,654671
315. Thorogood M, Mann J, Murphy M, Vessey M: Fatal stroke and use of oral contraceptives: finding from case-control study. Am J Epidemiol 136, 1992, 35-45
316. Tietjen GB: The relationship of migraine and stroke. Neuroepidemiology 19, 2000, 13-13
317. Toni D, Fiorelli M, De Mickele M, Bastanello S, Sacchetti ML, Montinaro E, Zanette EM, Argentino C: Clinical and prognosis correlates of stroke subtype mist diagnosis within 12 hours from onset. Stroke 26, 1995, 1837-1840
318. Truelsen T, Lidenstrom E, Boysen G: Comparison of probability of stroke between Copenhagen City earth Study and the Framingam Study. Stroke 25, 1994, 802-807
319. Tsuda Y, Saton K, Kitadai M, Takahashi T: Hemorheologic profiles of plasma fibrinogen and blood viscosity from silent to acute and chronic cerebral infarction. J Neurol Sci 147, 1997,49-54
320. Tuomilehto J, Rastenyte D, Jousilahti P, Sarti C, Varianainen E: Diabetes mellitus as a risk factor for death from stroke. Prospective study of the middle-aged Finish population. Stroke 27, 1996, 210-215
321. Tzourio C, Bousser MG: Migraine and risk of cerebral infarction. Rev Neurol156, 2000, 47-56
322. Tzourio C, Tehindrazanarivelo A, Iglesias S, Alpetrovitch A, Chedru F, D'Anglejan-Chatillon J, Bousser MG: Case-control study of migraine and risk of ischemic stroke in young women. BMJ 310, 1995, 830-833
323. Tzourio C, Bousser MG: Migraine: a risk factor for ischemic stroke in young women. Stroke 28, 1997, 2569-2570
324. Tzourio C, Kittner SJ, Bousser MG, Alperovitch A: Migraine and stroke in young women. Cephalgia 20,2000, 190-199

325. UK Prospective Diabetes Study (UKPDS) Group. Intensive blood-glucose control with sulphonylureas or insulin compared with conventional treatment with risk of complications in patients with type 2 diabetes (UKPDS 33). Lancet 352, 1998,837-853
326. Vaitkus PT: Left ventricular mural thrombus and risk of embolic stroke after acute myocardial infarction. J Cardiovasc Risk 2, 1995, 103-106
327. Venneri A, Caffara P: Transient autobiographic amnesia: EEG and single-photon emission CT evidence of an organic etiology. Neurology
328. 50,1998,186-191
329. Verdecchia P, Schillaci G, Bargioni C, Cuicci A, Gattobiogio R, zampi I, Porcellati C: Prognostic value of a new electrocardiographic method for diagonosis of left venricular hypertrophy in essential hypertension. J Am Coli Cardiol 31,1998,383-390
330. Vincent M, Cartier R, Privat P, Benzonu D, Samani NJ, Sassard J: Mayor cardiovascular risk factors in Lyon hypertensive rats. A correlation analysis in a segregation population. J Hypertens 14,1996,469-474
331. Viriyavejakul A, Senanarong V, Prayoonwiwat N, Praditsuwan R, Chaisevikul R, Poungvarin N: Epidemiology of stroke in the elderly in Tailand. J Med Assoc Thai 81,1998,497-505
332. Vohra EA, Ahmed WU, Ali M: Aetiology and prognostic factors of patients admitted for stroke. J Park Med Assoc 50,2000,234-236
333. Wang TO, Wu CC, Lee YT: Myocardial stunning after cerebral infarction. Int J Cardiol 58, 1997, 308-311
334. Wannamethee SG, Sharper AG, Whincup PH, Walker M:
335. Smoking cessation and the risk of stroke in middle-aged British men. JAMA 274,1995,155-160
336. Wannamethee SG, Sharper AG, Ebrahim S: HDL-Cholesterol, total cholesterol, and the risk of stroke in middle-aged British men. Stroke 31,2000,1882-1888
337. Weerasuriya N, Siribaddana S, Dissanayake A, Subasinghe Z, Wariyapola D, Fernando OJ: Long-term complications in newly diagnosed Sri Lankan
338. patients with type 2 diabetes mellitus. QJM 91, 1998, 439-443
339. Weir J, Murray GD, Dyken AG, Lees KR: Is hyperglycaemia an independent predictor of poor outcome after acute stroke? Results of a long-term follow-up study. BMJ 314, 1998, 1303-1306 311. Welch KM: Relationship of strike and migraine. Neurology 44, 1994, 33-36
340. Whisnant JP, Wiebers DO, O'Fallon WM, Sicks JD, Freye RL: A population-based model of risk factors for ischemic stroke: Rochester, Minnesota. Neurology 47, 1996, 1420-1428
341. Who Collaborative Study of Cardiovascular Disease and Steroid Hormone Contraception. Hemorrhagic stroke, overall stroke risk, and combined oral contraceptives: results of an International multicentre, case-control study. Lancet 348, 1996,505-510
342. Who Collaborative Study of Cardiovascular Disease and Steroid Hormone Contraception. Hemorrhagic stroke, overall stroke risk, and combined oral

contraceptives: results of an International multicentre, case-control study. Lancet 348, 1996,498-505
343. Wilson WP, Musella L, Short MJ: The electroencephalogram in dementia. Contemp-Neurol Ser 15, 1977, 205-221
344. Wilson PW, Hoeg JM, D'Agostino RB, Silbershatz H, Belanger AM, Poehmann H, O'leary D, Wolf PA: Cumulative effects of high cholesterol levels, high blood pressure, and cigarette smoking on carotid stenosis. N Engl J Med 337,1997,516-522
345. Witczak W, Banca S, Janiszewska A, Ginszt A,
346. Ziolkowska U, Bacmaga J: Cardiologic risk factors for stroke. Neurol Neurochir Pol 32, 1998,31-37
347. Wolf PA: An overview of the epidemiology of stroke. Stroke 21,1990,4-6
348. Wolf P: Contribution of epidemiology to the prevention of stroke. Circulation 88,1993,2471-2478
349. Wolf P, Abbot R, Kannel W: Atrial fibrillation, a major contributor to stroke in the elderly: The Framingam Study. Arch Intern Med 147, 1987, 1561-1564
350. Wolf P, Belanger A, D'Agostino R: Management of risk factors. In: A. Barnett, Hachinski (eds.) *Neurologic Clinics. Cerebrallschemia: Treatment and Prevention,* W. B. Sanders Company, Philadelphia, London, Torino, Montreal, Sydney, Tokio 177,1992, p. 191
351. Wolf PA, Kannel WB, Verter J: Current status of risk factors for stroke. Neurol Clinics 1, 1983, 317-343
352. Wolf P, Kannel W, Cupples LA, D'Agostino R: Epidemiologic appraisal of hypertension and stroke risk. In: A. Bes, G. Gerald (eds.) *Cerveau et hypertension arterielle,* Masson, Paris, New York, Barcelona, Milan, Mexico, Sao Paolo, 1986, pp. 184-196
353. Wolf P, Kannel W, Cupples LA, D'Agostino R: Risk factor interaction in cardiovascular disease. In: A. Furlan (ed.) *The Heart and Stroke.* Springer Verlag, London, Berlin, Heidelberg, New York, Tokyo, 1987, pp.331-355
354. Wooward M, Rumley A, Tunstaall-Pedoe H, Lowe GO: Associations of blood rheology and interleuckin-6 with cardiovascular risk factors and
355. prevalent cardiovascular disease. Br J Haematol1 04, 1999, 246-257
356. Xu WL, Geng GY, Wang PS: A study of risk factors of cerebral hemorrhage in women. No To Shinkei 46, 1994, 1143-1145
357. Yamamoto M, Egusa G, Hara H, Yamakido M: Association of intraabdominal fat and carotid atherosclerosis in non-obese middle-aged men with normal glucose tolerance. Int Jobes Relat Metab Disord 21, 1997,948-951
358. Yamanouchi H, Nagura H, Mizutani T, Matsushita S, Esaki Y: Embolic brain infarction in nonrehumatic atrial fibrillation: a clinicopathologic study in the elderly. Neurol 48, 1997, 1593-1597
359. Yamashita K, Kobayashi S, Yamaguchi S, Koide H: Cigarette smoking and silent brain infarction in normal adults. Intern Med 35, 1995, 704-706
360. Yokoyama E, Nagata K, Hirata Y, Satoh Y, Watahiki Y, Yuha H: Correlation of EEG activities between slow-wave sleep and wakefulness in patients with supratentoral stroke. Brain Topogr 8, 1996, 269-273

361. Yoshida M, Nakamura Y, Higashikawa M, Kinoshita M: Predictors of ischemic stroke in nonrheumatic atrial fibrillation. Int J Cardiol56, 1996,61-70
362. Yuan Z, Bowlin S, Eistadter D, Cebul RD, Conners AR, Rimm AA: Atrial fibrillation as a risk factor for stroke: a retrospective cohort study of hospitalized Medicare beneficiaries. Am J Public Health 88, 1998, 395-400
363. Yusuf HR, Giles WH, Anda RF, Casper ML: Impact of multiple risk factor profiles on
364. determining cardiovascular disease risk. Prev Med 27, 1998, 1-9
365. Zabsorne P, Yomeogo A, Millogo A, Dyemkouma FX, Durand G: Risk and severity factors in cerebrovascular accidents in west African Blacks of Burkina Faso. Med Trop (Mars) 57,1997, 147152
366. Zeitoun K, Carr BR: Is there increased risk of stroke associated with oral contraceptives? Drug Saf 20, 1999,467-473
367. Zodpey SP, Tiwari RR, Kalkarni HR: Risk factors for hemorrhagic stroke: a case-control study. Public Health 114, 2000, 177-182
368. Zuber M, Mas JL: Epidemiology of cerebrovascular accidents. Rev Neurol, Paris 148, 1992,243-255
369. Zurek R, Schieman-Delgado J, Froescher W, Niedermeyer E: Frontal intermittment rhythmical delta activity and anterior bradyarhytmia. Clin Electroencephalogr 16, 1985, 1-10.

ABBREVIATIONS USED IN THE MONOGRATH

AH	Arterial hypertension
ACS	Asymptomatic carotid stenoses
DSG	Doppler sonography
EEG	Electroencephalogram
ECG	Electrocardiogram
IHD	Ischemic heart disease
CT	Computed tomography of the brain
CI	Cerebral infarction
CVD	Cerebrovascular disease
CVDs	Cerebrovascular disorders
NAF	Non-rheumatic atrial fibrillation
ICCD	Ischemic cerebral circulatory disorders
TIA'S	Transient ischemic attacks
AF	Atrial fibrillation
PAF	Paroxysmal atrial fibrillation
RF	Risk factor
SPECT	Single photon emission computed tomography
CAF	Chronic atrial fibrillation
CRF	Cerebrovascular risk factor
BMI	Body mass index
OR	Option ratio
RR	Relative risk

LaVergne, TN USA
21 May 2010
183521LV00001B/60/P